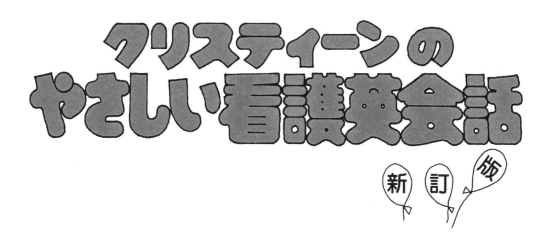

クリスティーンのやさしい看護英会話

新訂版

知念クリスティーン
元九州大学助教授

上瀧真紀恵
ウォルデン英語教室主宰

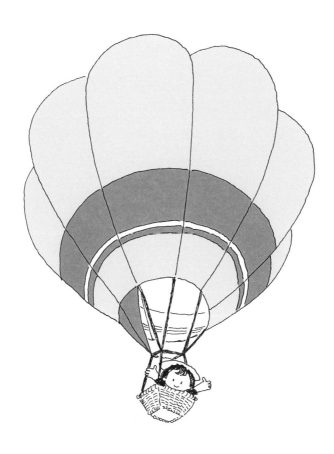

医学書院

クリスティーンのやさしい看護英会話

発　行　1995 年 4 月 15 日　第 1 版第 1 刷
　　　　2022 年 10 月 15 日　第 1 版第 30 刷
　　　　2023 年 11 月 1 日　新訂版第 1 刷©

著　者　知念クリスティーン・上瀧真紀恵

発行者　株式会社　医学書院
　　　　代表取締役　金原　俊
　　　　〒113-8719　東京都文京区本郷 1-28-23
　　　　電話　03-3817-5600(社内案内)

印刷・製本　アイワード

ISBN978-4-260-05250-4

謝辞

この本の完成にあたって直接，あるいは間接的にご協力いただいた皆様にお礼を申し上げます．

本書を医学書院に紹介してくださった野村光子氏，提案，批評，励ましをいただいた Diana Lee 氏，情報と知識を提供していただいた Steve Sabotta 氏，Emergency English を示していただいた Jay Kilpatrick 氏，医療関連の情報，知識をいただいた医師の玉城欣也先生，澤村經先生，恒吉香保子先生に厚くお礼申し上げます．

Acknowledgements

There are many people whom I want to thank for their help, either direct or indirect in the completion of this book :

Mitsuko Nomura, for introducing my book to IGAKU-SHOIN ; Diana Lee, for her encouragement, suggestions and criticisms ; Steve Sabotta, for his input and for coming to my house at midnight to fix the keyboard of my computer ; Jay Kilpatrick, for teaching me "Emergency English"; and Dr. Kinya Tamaki, Dr. Osamu Sawamura, and Dr. Kahoko Tsuneyoshi for their assistance with the medical aspects.

1995 年 2 月
Christine Lee Chinen
上瀧　真紀恵

新訂版に添えて

本書の著者，知念クリスティーンが闘病の末に亡くなって 20 年余りが経ちました．今回，クリスティーンの思いを引き継ぎつつ，イラストや語句を一部アップデートし，同時に電子書籍化を行い，音声データもダウンロードできるようにし，新訂版といたしました．

在留外国人が急増し，看護師が外国人の患者さんと接する機会がますます増える中で英語が駆使できれば，日本語が得意ではない患者さんにも安心感を与え，適切な看護を提供できるでしょう．そのための第一歩として，新しくなった本書が皆さんのお役に立てることをクリスティーンと共に願ってやみません．

2023 年 10 月
上瀧　真紀恵

CONTENTS

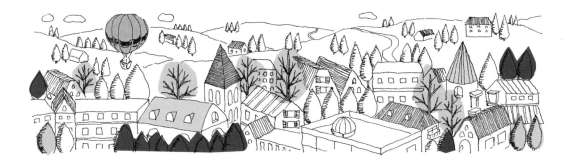

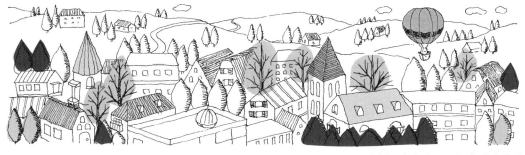

表紙・本文イラスト/加藤由美子

このテキストで学習されるみなさんへ

　このテキストは，看護学校の学生のために書かれた英会話の教科書です．もちろん，現場スタッフにも使っていただけるテキストです．外国人である著者が，日本で患者として何度も通院，入院をしたときの経験をもとに書かれています．慣れない国で病気になってしまった外国人にとって，意思の疎通をはかろうと懸命になってくれる看護師や英語を話す医師は，病気や慣れない環境での不安や恐怖を軽くしてくれるありがたい存在です．

　看護師と患者のやりとりは，大きく2つのタイプに分けられます．1つは患者への質問，もう1つは患者に指示や説明をすることです．1年という短期間で，必ずしも流暢な英語を話せるようになる必要はありません．看護師の日常の業務に必要な英語はかぎられていますから，それに慣れ親しむことができればよいと思います．

　日本在住の外国人が少なくない今，医療スタッフにとって，外国人患者と意思の疎通をはかれることは，重要な責務の1つになろうとしています．そのためにも，皆さんには大いにこのテキストを利用していただきたいと思います．

　Unit 1 に出てくる Emergency English は，このテキストの中で最も重要な学習ポイントであり，皆さんが英語で意思の疎通をはかる上で，心強い味方となってくれます．患者と話すときでも，外国旅行の際でも，"Can you please speak more slowly?" や "Say that again, please." などを知っていれば，会話をいくらかでも前に進めることができます．

　ですから，Emergency English は，暗記して授業中に先生に対して，あるいは他の学生との会話練習のときにどんどん使って，ぜひとも自分のものにしてください．そうすることによって，少しくらい間違えても，たどたどしい英語であっても，自分は英語で意思の疎通ができるのだという自信をもてるようになります．

　このテキストにある のついた頁(単語やフレーズ)については，ネイティブスピーカーの発音があり，それを聞いて学習を進めるようになっています．ネイティブスピーカーの発音は医学書院のウェブサイト(https://www.igaku-shoin.co.jp/book/detail/113474/appendix)から無料でダウンロードできます(ID：kangoeikaiwa, PW：christine)．

　ネイティブスピーカーによる正しい発音を繰り返し聞き，それを真似ることで正しい英語が身につくはずです．また Audio を利用することで，グループでの学習や自主学習ができます．

テキストの構成と使い方を簡単に説明しましょう．

DIALOG

　最初はテキストを見ないで，Audio を何度か聞いて場面の雰囲気をつかみながら，内容の理解に努めます．ある程度内容の理解ができたところで初めてテキストを見て，わからなかった部分をチェックします．すべて理解できたら，もう一度 Audio を聞き，発音，イントネーションを耳になじませ，一文ずつ繰り返して言ってみます．最後にパートナー役を決めてテキストを見ないで会話練習をします．

CHECKPOINT

　特に覚えておきたい表現なので，やはり Audio で正確な発音を聞いて確認した上で，スピーキング練習をしましょう．

MEDICAL TERMS

　専門的なものも多くのせていますが，Audio をフル活用してできるだけ耳になじませてほしいものです．また，現場スタッフの場合は，各自の現場で必要と思われるものを選んで覚えればよいでしょう．

PRACTICE

　さまざまなタイプの練習問題がありますが，その多くがクラス，あるいはグループで行うものです．独学でできる部分もありますが，できれば2人以上で練習すると効果的です．特にロールプレイは，練習すればするほど効果があるので，テキストの設問以外にも独自に状況を設定して練習を行うようにするとよいでしょう．

GAME

　Unit 2 以降には Unit の最後にゲームを設けています．ゲームで英単語やフレーズを口にしたり書いたりすることで楽しく英語を学べるようにしています．時間がある限り，クラスでやってみてください．

　このテキストは，たくさんのゲームやイラストで楽しく英会話の学習ができるように工夫されています．皆さんが楽しみながらこのテキストを使い，また楽しみながら英語を使って会話をされることを願ってやみません．

Christine Lee Chinen

上瀧　真紀恵

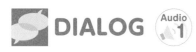**DIALOG**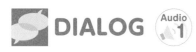

Foreigner : Excuse me. Could you tell me the way to St. Luke's Hospital?

Japanese : Pardon? Can you please speak more slowly?

Foreigner : Could you tell me the way to St. Luke's Hospital?

Japanese : I'm sorry. I don't know.

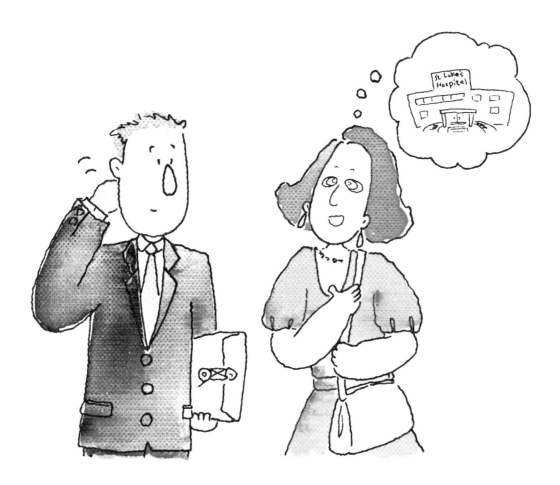

foreigner：外国人　　Excuse me：（人にものを尋ねるときや，ちょっと通してほしいときなどの）すみません　　Pardon (me)：（問い返すときの）すみません，（小さな過失，例えばげっぷやおならをしたときの）失礼しました　slowly：ゆっくりと

✓ CHECKPOINT

1. 相手の言っていることが聞き取れない，あるいはわからないとき

   Excuse me?
   Pardon (me)?
   Can you please speak more slowly (loudly)?
   Say that again, please.

2. もう一度，あるいはゆっくり言ってもらってもわからないとき

   I don't understand.

3. 質問の答えがわからないとき

   I don't know.

4. 答えがすぐに出てこないとき，「えーと…」

   Let me see…….
   Well…….

5. 答えたいけれども，それを英語で言えないとき

   I know the answer, but can't say it in English.

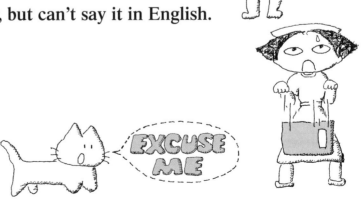

---

emergency：非常の場合，緊急　　loudly：大きな声で

6. 単語の意味がわからないとき

What does <u>occupation</u> mean?

7. 単語の綴りがわからないとき

How do you spell <u>Macintosh</u>?

 It's M-A-C-I-N-T-O-S-H.

8. 相手の言ったことを確認したいとき

Did you say <u>right or left</u>?

 I said left.

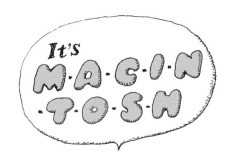

9. 英語で何というのか知りたいとき

How do you say *kouketsuatsu*(高血圧) in English?

 Hypertension.

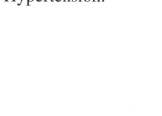

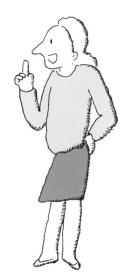

✎ PRACTICE Speaking & Listening

先生が質問しますから，"Emergency English" を使って会話をしてみましょう．

---

occupation：職業 mean：意味する spell：綴る Macintosh：マッキントッシュ

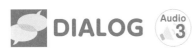

Unit 2 — Where are you from?

DIALOG Audio 3

Masako : Hello, my name is Masako Sato. What's your name?

Brian : I'm Brian Daly. What do you do?

Masako : I'm a nurse. What do you do?

Brian : I'm a baseball player. Where are you from?

Masako : I'm from Hiroshima in Japan. Where do you come from?

Brian : I come from Seattle, Washington.

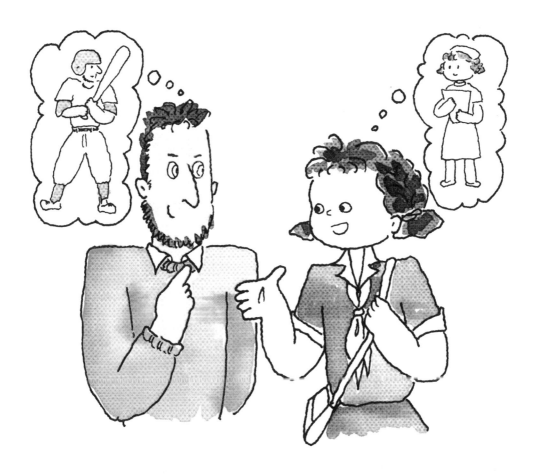

be from, come from：〜の出身である

Unit **2**

✓ CHECKPOINT

自己紹介のときなどに使う，基本的な質問と答え方を覚えましょう.

1. お名前は？

What's your name?

May I ask your name, please?

My name is <u>Masako Sato</u>.

I'm <u>Brian Daly</u>.

2. お仕事は何ですか.

What do you do?

What's your occupation?

I'm <u>a nurse</u>.

3. 出身地はどこですか.

Where are you from?

Where do you come from?

I'm from <u>Sendai</u>.

I come from <u>Seattle, Washington</u>.

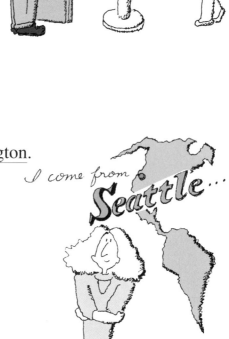

4. どこで生まれましたか.

Where were you born?

What's your birthplace?

I was born in <u>Tokyo</u>.

5. どこに住んでいますか.

Where do you live?

I live in <u>Kanda</u>.

---

occupation：職業　　be born：生まれる　　birthplace：出生地

6. 誰といっしょに住んでいますか.

Who do you live with?

    I live alone.

    I live with my <u>family</u>.

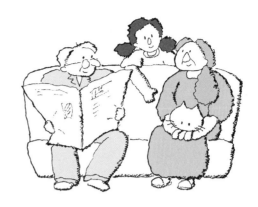

7. あなたの姓（名）はどう綴りますか.

How do you spell <u>your last (first) name</u>?

    It's S-U-Z-U-K-I (M-A-R-I-K-O).

8. 何歳ですか. *

How old are you?
May I ask how old you are?

    I'm <u>eighteen</u> years old.

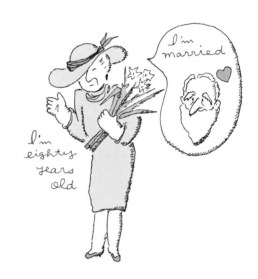

9. 結婚していますか，独身ですか. *

Are you married or single?
What's your marital status?

    I'm married (single).
    I'm divorced.

＊CHECKPOINT 8,9 は，看護師として質問するのはかまいませんが，一般の会話では，会ったばかりの人に質問すると失礼になりますから気をつけましょう.

10. 兄弟，姉妹は何人いますか.

How many brothers and sisters do you have?

    I have <u>two brothers and one sister</u>.

---

alone：1人で   last name：姓   first name：名   how old：何歳
marital status：婚姻区分   married：既婚，結婚している   single：独身
divorced：離婚して   how many：(数を聞くとき，数えられる場合)いくつ，何人

11. 趣味は何ですか.

What is your hobby?

My hobby is <u>playing the piano</u>.

12. (一番)好きなスポーツは何ですか.

What sport do you like (best／most)?
What is your favorite sport?

I like <u>baseball</u> (best／most).

My favorite sport is <u>baseball</u>.

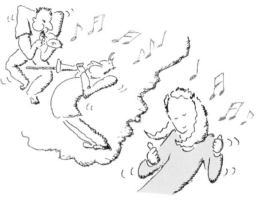

13. どんな音楽が好きですか.

What kind of music do you like?

I like <u>jazz</u>.

hobby：趣味	most：最も，一番	favorite：大好きな	kind of～：～の種類

PRACTICE Speaking

英語で自己紹介をしましょう. 自分の名前, 出身地, どこで誰と住んでいるか, 家族構成, 趣味について話してください.

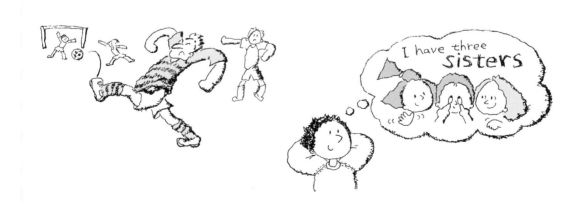

📖 PRACTICE Speaking & Listening

2人一組になって次の質問をやりとりし，相手の答えを書き取りましょう．

1. How do you spell your first name?

2. Who do you live with?

3. Where were you born?

4. What sport do you like most?

5. How many brothers and sisters do you have?

6. Who's your favorite singer?

7. What's your hobby?

first name：名前(姓名の名)　　singer：歌手

🎤 GAME Name Game　どこまで覚えられる？

順番を決め，最初の人から自分の名前と好きなものを言っていきます．2人目の人からは，前の人が言ったすべての名前と好きなものを覚えていて，言わなければなりません．最後に近い人ほど大変なゲームです．

例) Student 1：My name is Kyoko and I like apples.

Student 2：Her name is Kyoko and she likes apples.

My name is Masao and I like baseball.

Student 3：Her name is Kyoko and she likes apples.

His name is Masao and he likes baseball.

My name is Chie and I like J-pop.

……

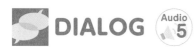

Unit 3
Could you tell me your address, please?

DIALOG Audio 5

Masako : I'd like to ask you some questions.

Ms. Wilson : Yes?

Masako : Could you tell me your address, please?

Ms. Wilson : 28-23 Hongo 1-chome Bunkyo-ku, Tokyo.

Masako : What's your telephone number?

Ms. Wilson : 03-3817-5600.

Masako : What is your date of birth?

Ms. Wilson : July 15, 1998.

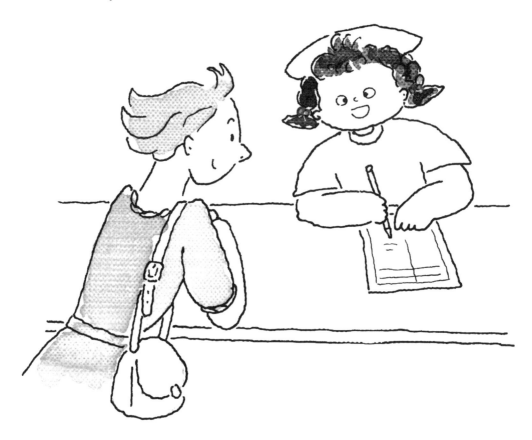

---

address：住所　　question：質問　　telephone (phone) number：電話番号
date of birth：誕生日

✓ CHECKPOINT

●ていねいな質問のしかたを覚えましょう.

1. コーヒーが飲みたいのですが(「〜したい」のていねいな言い方).

   I'd (I would) like to <u>have a cup of coffee.</u>

2. あなたの名前を教えていただけますか.

   Could (Would) you tell me your <u>name</u>, **please?**

      Yes, it's Mary Smith.

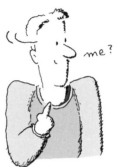

3. 質問してもよろしいですか.

   May (Can) I <u>ask you some questions?</u>

      Sure.

4. 体重はどのくらいありますか.

   How much do you weigh?

      I weigh <u>52 kilograms</u>.

5. 身長はどのくらいありますか.

   How tall are you?

      I'm <u>162 centimeters</u> tall.

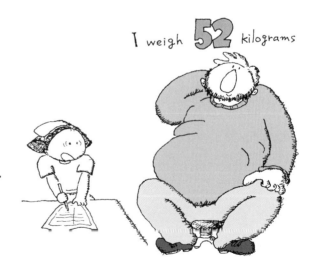

---

a cup of coffee：1杯のコーヒー　　how much：(量を聞くとき, 数えられない場合)どのくらい
weigh：〜の重さがある　　kilogram：キログラム　　tall：〜の高さがある
centimeter：センチメートル

Unit 3

●住所，電話番号の書き方，読み方を覚えましょう． Audio 7

●例えば

〒980-0004　宮城県仙台市青葉区宮町 2 丁目 5-20

山田アパート 305 号

佐藤　雅子　様

●英語の書き方

Ms. Masako Sato

305 Yamada Apt.

5-20 Miyamachi 2-chome Aoba-ku,

Sendai, Miyagi, Japan　〒980-0004

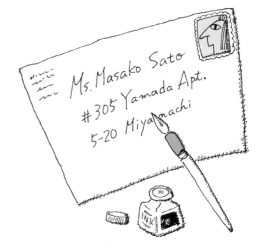

●英語の読み方

Ms. Masako Sato

three zero five, Yamada Apartment,

five dash twenty Miyamachi two-chome Aoba-ku,

Sendai, Miyagi, Japan

postal code, nine eight zero dash zero zero zero four

●電話番号の読み方

03-3817-5600

zero three, three eight one seven,

five six zero zero

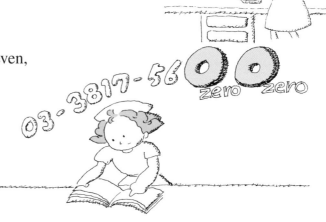

---

apartment：アパート　　postal code：郵便番号

●**18**

●日付や順序を表わす数を「序数」といいます.

序数 1 から 31 の言い方を覚えましょう.

1st first	11th eleventh	21st twenty-first
2nd second	12th twelfth	22nd twenty-second
3rd third	13th thirteenth	23rd twenty-third
4th fourth	14th fourteenth	24th twenty-fourth
5th fifth	15th fifteenth	25th twenty-fifth
6th sixth	16th sixteenth	26th twenty-sixth
7th seventh	17th seventeenth	27th twenty-seventh
8th eighth	18th eighteenth	28th twenty-eighth
9th ninth	19th nineteenth	29th twenty-ninth
10th tenth	20th twentieth	30th thirtieth
		31st thirty-first

●日付, 年号の書き方, 読み方を覚えましょう.

●書き方	●読み方
June 3, 1982	June third, nineteen eighty-two
April 15, 1995	April fifteenth, nineteen ninety-five

1975	nineteen seventy-five
2000	two thousand
2005	two thousand five
2036	twenty thirty-six

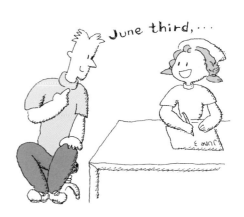

PRACTICE Pronunciation

1. Audio のあとについて数字の発音練習をしましょう. (Audio 10)

    1）12 20   2）13 30   3）14 40   4）15 50

    5）16 60   6）17 70   7）18 80   8）19 90

    9）100   10）111   11）250   12）1000

2. Audio のあとについて曜日，月の発音練習をしましょう. (Audio 11)

1）曜日

Sunday／Monday／Tuesday／Wednesday／Thursday／Friday／Saturday

2）月

January／February／March／April／May／June／July／August／September／
October／November／December

PRACTICE Listening

1. 聞こえたほうの数字を○でかこんでください. (Audio 12)

    1） 14   40   2） 70   17   3）12 20   4） 90   19

    5） 11   101   6） 15   50   7）18 80   8）160   116

    9）111   121   10）201   210

2. Audio をよく聞いて，年月日を書き取りましょう. (Audio 13)

例）January first, nineteen forty-four；1944 年 1 月 1 日

    1）_____   2）_____   3）_____

    4）_____   5）_____

3. Audio をよく聞いて，電話番号を書き取りましょう. (Audio 14)

    1）_____   2）_____   3）_____

    4）_____   5）_____

PRACTICE Speaking & Listening

5人のクラスメートに名前，住所，電話番号を英語で聞いて書き取りましょう．

name	address	phone No.
	〒	
	〒	
	〒	
	〒	
	〒	

GAME Bingo Game　ビンゴゲーム

BINGO の各列を下に示した数字の中から自分の好きな数字でうめます．次に先生が数字をアトランダムに読み上げますから，各列に読み上げられた数字があれば，その数字を×で消していきます．早く×が5つ並んだ人が勝ちです．

B : 1〜15　　I : 16〜30　　N : 31〜45　　G : 46〜60　　O : 61〜75

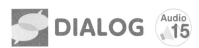

Unit 4
What department do you want to visit?

DIALOG Audio 15

Masako : Is this your first visit?

Ms. Smith : Yes, it is.

Masako : Do you have an insurance card?

Ms. Smith : No, I don't.

Masako : What department do you want to visit?

Ms. Smith : I want to go to dermatology.

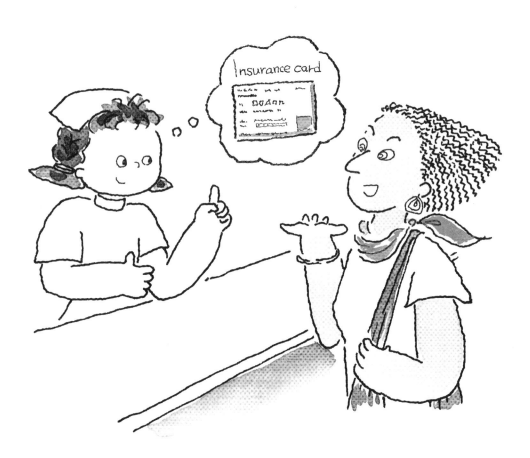

---

department：(診療)科　　visit：訪れる　　first visit：初診　　insurance card：保険証
dermatology：皮膚科

☑ CHECKPOINT

初診の患者が訪れたときに使う，基本的な質問を覚えましょう.

1. 初診ですか.

   Is this your first visit?

   > Yes, it is.／No, it isn't.

2. 保険証はお持ちですか.

   Do you have <u>an insurance card</u>?

   > Yes, I do.／No, I don't.

3. 保険証をお見せください.

   Please show me your <u>insurance card</u>.

4. 何科にかかりたいのですか.

   What department do you want to visit?

   > I want to visit <u>surgery</u>.

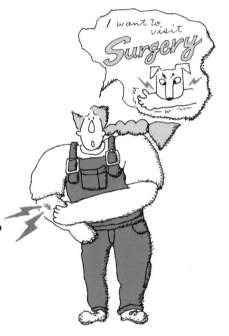

🩺 MEDICAL TERMS Departments 診療科名を覚えましょう.

internal medicine　内科	psychiatry　精神科
surgery　外科	neurology　神経科
orthopedics　整形外科	radiology　放射線科
pediatrics　小児科	anesthesiology　麻酔科
obstetrics／gynecology　産科／婦人科	dentistry　歯科
dermatology　皮膚科	cardiosurgery　心臓外科
urology　泌尿器科	ophthalmology (eye clinic)　眼科
neurosurgery　脳神経外科	otorhinolaryngology　耳鼻咽喉科 (ear, nose, & throat clinic : ENT)

Unit 4

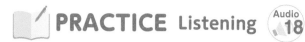 **PRACTICE** Listening Audio 18

Audio を聞いて，読み上げた順に番号をつけましょう.

( ) ophthalmology   ( ) anesthesiology

( ) orthopedics   ( ) pediatrics

( ) cardiosurgery   ( ) neurology

PRACTICE Role Play

2人一組になって，看護師役と患者役を決めます.

看護師役は患者役に質問してAの診療申込書に記入します．患者役はBのカードにある外国人になったつもりで看護師役の質問に答えてください.

診療申込書に記入し終わったら役割を交代して，患者役は今度はCのカードに記載された外国人になって練習しましょう.

A：診療申込書

⑪内	神	児	外	整	皮	泌	産婦	眼	耳	放	心外	歯
ふりがな ① 氏名							② 性別　男・女・他					
							③ 職業			④ 既婚・未婚		
⑤ 生年 月日	西暦　　　　　年　　　月　　　日 ⑥ 満(　　)歳						⑧ 勤務先電話番号 (　　　　)　　　－					
⑦ 現住所	〒　　　－						⑨ 電話番号(　　　)　　　－					
⑩ 出生地												

B：患者

NAME： *Nancy Wright*	**OCCUPATION：** *Singer*
SEX： *Female*	**AGE：** *39*
ADDRESS： *11-3 Kuromon 5-chome*	**MARITAL STATUS：** *Married*
Chuo-ku, Fukuoka 〒810-0055	
TELEPHONE： *(092)423-8095 (home)*	
(092)389-5829 (work)	
BIRTHDATE： *January 25, 1984*	**DEPARTMENT：** *Obstetrics／Gynecology*
BIRTHPLACE： *Orlando, Florida*	

C：患者

NAME： *John Carradyne*	**OCCUPATION：** *Student*
SEX： *Male*	**AGE：** *19*
ADDRESS： *24-8-101 Sendagi 4-chome*	**MARITAL STATUS：** *single*
Bunkyo-ku, Tokyo 〒113-0022	
TELEPHONE： *(03)3381-4367 (home)*	
BIRTHDATE： *September 9, 2004*	**DEPARTMENT：** *Surgery*
BIRTHPLACE： *Birmingham, England*	

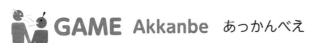

sex：性　　address：住所　　occupation：職業　　age：年齢　　marital status：婚姻区分

GAME Akkanbe　あっかんべえ

単語の綴りを覚えるためのゲームです．先生の指示に従って，ゲームで楽しみながら診療科名を覚えましょう．

Unit 5 Where is the X-ray department?

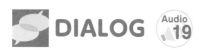

DIALOG Audio 19

Masako :	Ms. Lightfoot, please go to the X-ray department.
Ms. Lightfoot :	Where is the X-ray department?
Masako :	Go out of this office and turn right.
	Go straight up the hall and radiology is on the left.
Ms. Lightfoot :	I go out of this office and turn right, then I go
	straight up the hall and radiology is on the left.
Masako :	That's right.

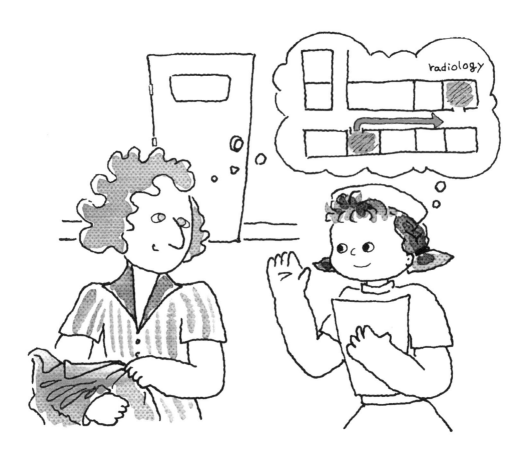

radiology

X-ray department, radiology：放射線科　　go out of〜：〜を出る　　office：診察室
turn：曲がる　　go straight up：まっすぐに進む　　hall：廊下　　then：それから，次に

CHECKPOINT 道順の尋ね方と答え方を覚えましょう.

●道順の尋ね方：すみませんが，放射線科にはどう行けばよいのでしょうか.

Excuse me, where is the X-ray department?

Could you tell me the way to the X-ray department?

Pardon me, how can I get to the X-ray department?

●道順を教える

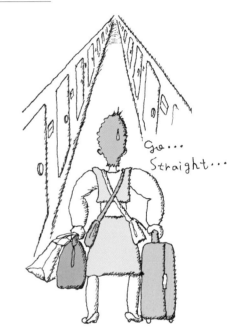

1. （廊下を）まっすぐに行ってください.

   Go straight (up the hall).

2. 右に（左に）行ってください.

   Turn right (left).

3. 1つめの角を右に（左に）曲がってください.

   Turn right (left) at the first corner.

4. 廊下を横切ってください.

   Cross the hall.

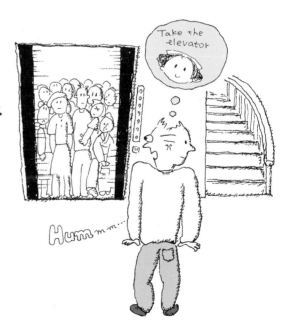

5. エレベーターで3階へ行ってください.

   Take the elevator to the 3rd floor.

●位置を教える

1. A は B のとなりにある.　A is next to B.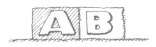

2. A は B と C の間にある.
   A is between B and C.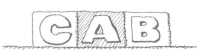

3. A は C の向かいにある.
   A is across from C.

4. A は左側にある.
   A is on the left.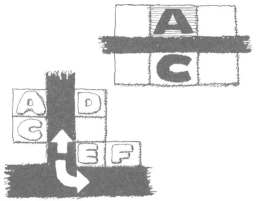

5. D は右側にある.
   D is on the right.

6. E は角にある.
   E is on the corner.

7. F は角を曲がったところにある.
   F is around the corner.

8. A は C を過ぎたところにある.
   A is just past C.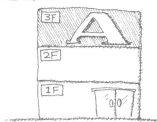

9. A は 3 階にある.　A is on the 3rd floor.

 PRACTICE Listening

　Audio の道案内を聞いて，下に示した場所を探し出し，次頁の病院の案内図に書き入れましょう．病院の入口 (entrance) からスタートしてください.

1. reception　　　　2. pharmacy　　　　3. surgery

4. urinalysis lab　　5. blood lab　　　　6. radiology

7. internal medicine　8. accounting　　　9. bank

10. hospital shop

---

reception：受付　　pharmacy：薬局　　surgery：外科　　urinalysis lab：尿検査室(lab は
laboratory の略)　　blood lab：血液検査室　　internal medicine：内科　　accounting：
会計　　bank：銀行

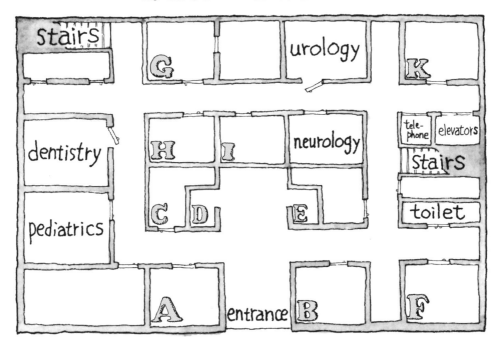

病院の案内図

PRACTICE Writing

完成した上の病院の案内図を見て，入口から次の場所までの行き方を書きましょう．

1. dentistry

2. neurology

3. elevators

4. urology

5. toilet

---

dentistry：歯科　　neurology：神経科　　elevator：エレベーター　　urology：泌尿器科
toilet：トイレ

GAME Hospital Map Game 院内オリエンテーリング

2人一組になります．2人とも，ところどころ名前のぬけた病院の案内図を持っています．Aの行きたい所はBの案内図にあり，Bの行きたい所はAの案内図に載っています．

お互いに行きたい場所を質問し，相手に入口からの道順を答えてもらって，案内図のどこにあるのか見つけて案内図を完成させてください．AとBがかわるがわる質問しないと見つからないようになっています．

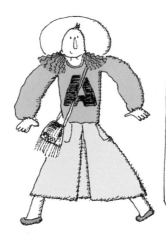

Aの行きたい場所
1. urology
2. surgery
3. pediatrics
4. gynecology
5. pharmacy

Aの案内図

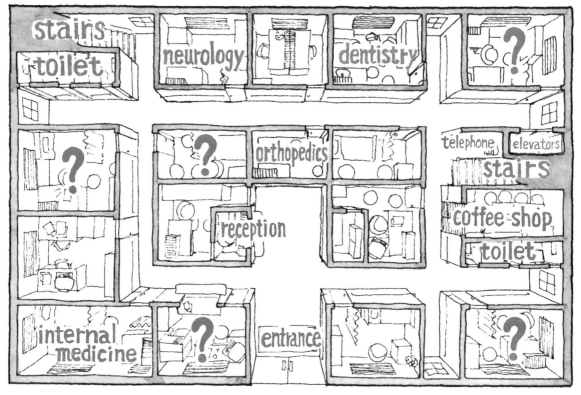

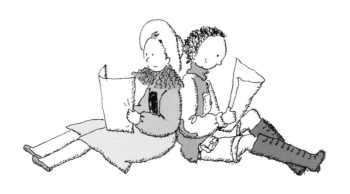

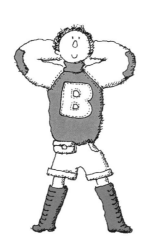

Bの行きたい場所
1. coffee shop
2. dentistry
3. orthopedics
4. neurology
5. internal medicine

Bの案内図

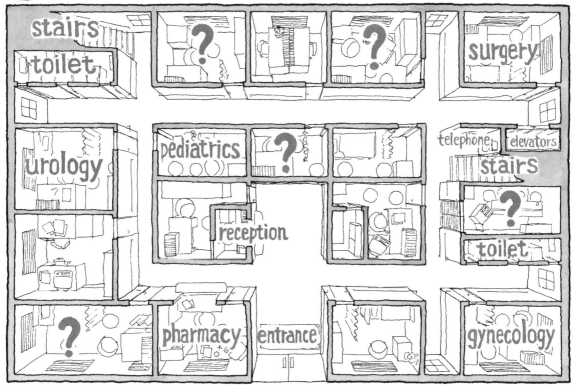

stairs
toilet
surgery
urology
pediatrics
telephone elevators
stairs
reception
toilet
pharmacy entrance
gynecology

Unit 6 What are your symptoms?

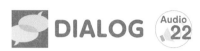

DIALOG Audio 22

Masako : Mr. Riley, what's your problem today?

Mr. Riley : I think I have a cold.

Masako : What are your symptoms?

Mr. Riley : I have a cough and I vomited last night.

Masako : How long have you been coughing?

Mr. Riley : For three days.

Masako : How many times did you vomit last night?

Mr. Riley : Twice.

Masako : Do you have a fever?

Mr. Riley : Yes. My temperature is 38.5℃.

Masako : Please wait. The doctor will see you in a few minutes.

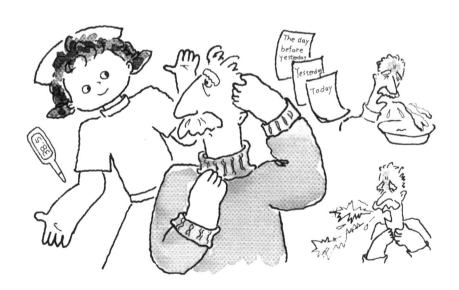

symptoms：症状，徴候　　problem：問題　　cold：かぜ　　cough：せき（をする）
vomit：嘔吐する　　last night：昨晩　　how long：どのくらいの期間　　for〜：〜（時間，期間）の間　　twice：2回　　fever：熱　　temperature：体温　　℃（degrees Celsius/centigrade）：摂氏〜度　　wait：待つ　　see：診察する　　a few：少しの，2, 3の

CHECKPOINT 症状の尋ね方を覚えましょう① Audio 23

1. どうしましたか.

   What's your problem today?
   What's the matter?

2. どんな症状ですか.

   What are your symptoms?
   What symptoms do you have?

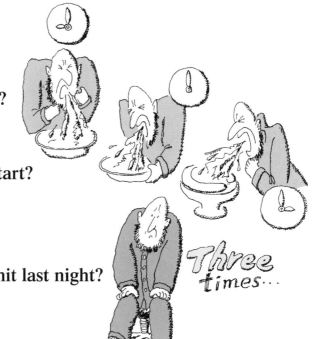

3. 下痢はいつ始まりましたか.

   When did the <u>diarrhea</u> first start?
   　　It started two days ago.

4. 昨夜, 何回嘔吐しましたか.

   How many times did you vomit last night?
   　　Three times.

5. 症状の続いている期間を聞く場合

   （持続している期間を尋ねる：How long have you＋過去分詞～?）

   ● 例 1）症状が動詞の場合

   せきはどのくらい続いていますか.

   How long have you been <u>coughing</u>?
   　　I've been coughing since yesterday (for two days).

   ● 例 2）症状が名詞の場合

   頭痛はどのくらい続いていますか.

   How long have you had <u>a headache</u>?
   　　I've had a headache since yesterday (for two days).

---

matter：問題　　diarrhea：下痢　　time(s)：～回　　since～：～(時刻, 日にちなど)から
headache：頭痛

🩺 MEDICAL TERMS Symptoms 症状と徴候の表現を覚えましょう. Audio 24

1. **Cold or flu symptoms** （かぜまたはインフルエンザの症状）

cough せき

runny nose 鼻水

stuffy nose 鼻づまり

headache 頭痛

fever 発熱

sneezing くしゃみ

sore throat のどの痛み

muscular aches 筋肉の痛み

shivers 寒気

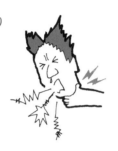

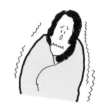

2. **Gastrointestinal symptoms** （消化器系の症状）

nausea 吐き気

vomiting (throwing up) 嘔吐

diarrhea 下痢

stomachache 胃痛（腹痛）

abdominal pain 腹痛

cramps けいれん, 急激な腹痛

upset stomach 胃の不調

gas ガス, おなら

constipation 便秘

burping げっぷ

vomiting of blood 吐血

appetite loss 食欲不振

bloody stool 血便

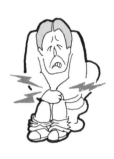

3. **Other symptoms and conditions** （その他の症状と状態）

pain 痛み

  severe pain 激しい痛み

  throbbing pain ずきずきする痛み

  stabbing (sharp) pain 刺すような痛み

  gripping pain しめつけられるような痛み

  dull pain 鈍痛

  soreness ひりひりする痛み

  chest pain 胸の痛み

  backache 背中の痛み, 腰痛

lower back pain 腰痛

toothache 歯痛

earache 耳痛

dizziness めまい

tiredness 疲れ

shortness of breath 息切れ

bleeding 出血

itching かゆみ

eruption, rash, spots 発疹, 皮疹

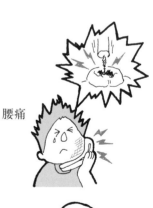

inflammation　炎症	menstruation　月経
numbness　しびれ	lump　しこり
pregnancy　妊娠	hardness of hearing　難聴
swelling　むくみ	something is stuck in one's throat
palpitations　動悸	何かが喉につまった（状態）
cold sweat　冷汗	nosebleed　鼻血
insomnia, trouble sleeping　不眠	ringing in the ears (tinnitus)　耳鳴り
convulsions　ひきつけ	eye discharge　目やに

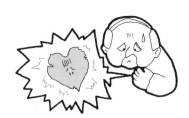 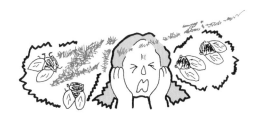

4．Usage（症状の訴え方） Audio 25

1）I have <u>a cold</u>.

　a cough/a runny nose/a fever/a sore throat/a backache/a headache/a toothache/
　an upset stomach/a rash on my～（身体の部分）/an earache/chest pain/gas/diarrhea/
　pain in my～（身体の部分）/cramps/something stuck in my throat

2）I am <u>nauseous</u>.

　sneezing/dizzy/tired/constipated/bleeding/pregnant

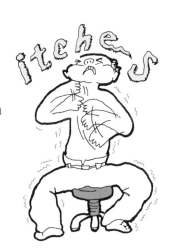

3）I feel <u>numbness in my left foot</u>（身体の部分）.

　pain in my <u>knee</u>（身体の部分）/dizzy/tired/short of breath

4）My <u>arm</u>（身体の部分） itches.

5）I vomited three times last night.

　I have been vomiting since last night.

人体各部については Unit 7 の p.42 を参照してください.

PRACTICE Writing 1

それぞれの絵に，その症状や状態を表す英語を書きましょう．

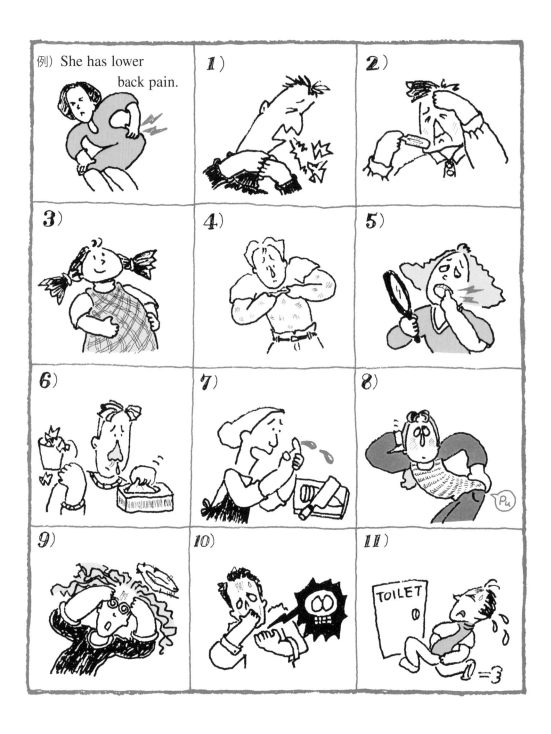

例）She has lower back pain.

1)

2)

3)

4)

5)

6)

7)

8)

9)

10)

11)

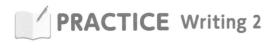

PRACTICE Writing 2

下のような症状や状態のときは，どの診療科に行ったらよいのでしょうか．適当な診療科名を
クロスワードに書きこみましょう．

ACROSS

1. My baby has a cough and a fever.

3. My eyes are itchy.

7. I have a rash.

8. I'm pregnant.

9. I need to have a chest X-ray.

10. I cut my hand on some glass.

11. I have a bladder infection.

DOWN

2. I have a stomachache, nausea and diarrhea.

4. I have a sore throat.

5. I have a toothache.

6. I have a terrible pain in my lower back.

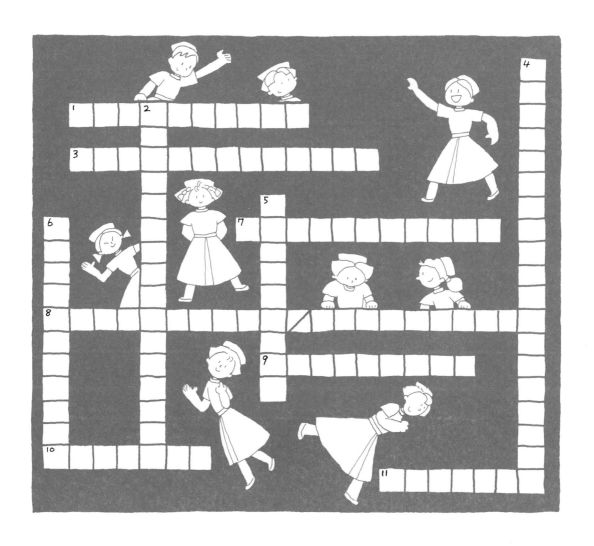

PRACTICE Role Play

　2人一組になって，看護師役と患者役を決めます．

　看護師役は，患者の名前と症状を聞いて A のカードの空欄をうめてください．患者役は，B の
カードにある外国人になったつもりで看護師役の質問に答えてください．

　カードに記入し終わったら役割を交代して，患者役は，今度は C のカードに記載された外国人
になって繰り返し練習しましょう．

A :

氏名　_____

症状　_____

期間　_____

B :

Name :　*Karen Storm*

Problem :　*I've been coughing and*
　　　　　　 I've had a fever.

How long : *for 3 days.*

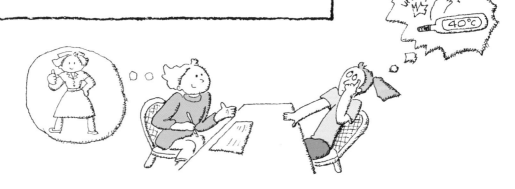

C:

Name : *Carole Gonzalez*

Problem : *I've had a headache and dizziness.*

How long : *for one week.*

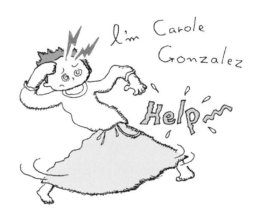

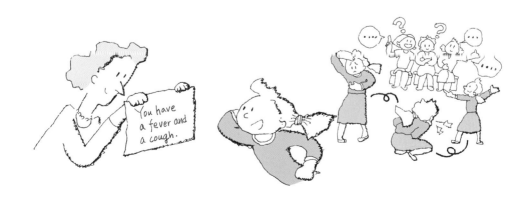

GAME What's the Matter? どこが悪いのでしょう？

　グループの中の1人に，先生からある症状や状態が告げられます．その人はグループのメンバーに，告げられた症状や状態を身ぶり手ぶりで表現し，ほかのメンバーはそれを見て，どんな症状かを当てます．

Unit 7 Where does it hurt?

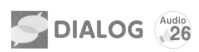 DIALOG Audio 26

Masako : Hello, Mr. Jordan. What's the problem today?

Mr. Jordan : I hurt my back and it's very painful.

Masako : Where does it hurt?

Mr. Jordan : Here.

Masako : Is it getting worse?

Mr. Jordan : Yes, it is.

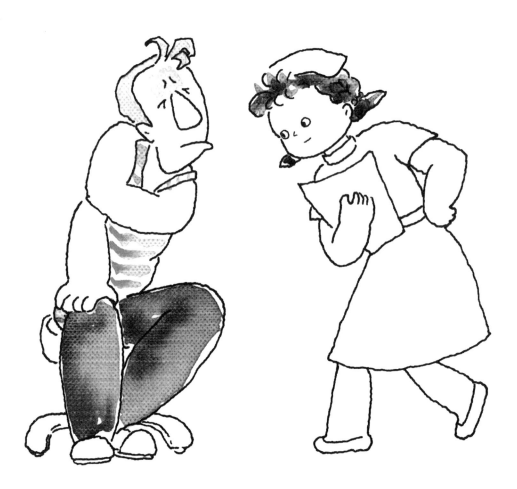

hurt：痛む，痛める，けがをする　　back：背中　　painful：痛い　　get worse：悪くなる

1. どこが痛みますか.

   Where does it hurt?

   Where is the pain?

   　　Here.

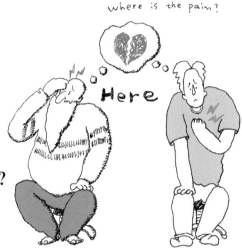

2. どんな痛みですか.

   What kind of pain is it?

   　　It's a sharp (dull／severe) pain.

3. いつ(脚を)ケガしましたか.

   When did you hurt <u>yourself</u> (your leg)?

   　　<u>This morning</u>.

4. どのようにしてケガをしましたか.

   How did you hurt yourself?

   　　I <u>hurt myself playing golf</u>.

5. 悪くなっていますか.

   Is it getting worse?

   　　Yes, it is.／No, it isn't.

   答えが Yes の場合；急速にですか，徐々にですか.

   Quickly or gradually?

   　　Gradually.

6. 何かほかの症状はありますか.

   Do you have any other symptoms?

   　　No, I don't.

   　　Yes, I have a pain here, too.

---

pain：痛み　　here：ここ　　sharp：刺すような　　dull：鈍い　　severe：激しい
quickly：急速に，どんどん　　gradually：徐々に，だんだん　　other：ほかの

Unit 7

♥ MEDICAL TERMS Parts of the Body

人体各部の名称を覚えましょう.

● 人体外部　External Body Parts

head　頭	armpit　腋窩	hip　股関節，左右の腰部
hair　髪	arm　腕	buttock　殿部
face　顔	elbow　肘	genitals　性器
forehead　額	wrist　手首	penis　陰茎
cheek　頬	hand　手	testicles　睾丸
chin　顎	palm　手のひら	anus　肛門
eye　目	finger　手の指	leg　脚
eyebrow　眉毛	thumb　親指	thigh　大腿
nose　鼻	nail　爪	knee　膝
mouth　口	skin　皮膚	calf　ふくらはぎ
lip　唇，口唇	chest　胸	ankle　足首，くるぶし
tooth　歯	breast　乳房	foot　足
tongue　舌	abdomen　腹	heel　かかと
ear　耳	back　背中	sole　足の裏
neck　首，頸	lower back　腰	toe　足の指
shoulder　肩	waist　ウエスト	

● 人体内部　Internal Body Parts

brain　脳	stomach　胃	large intestine　大腸
throat　咽喉	liver　肝臓	colon　結腸
tonsils　扁桃腺	spleen　脾臓	rectum　直腸
muscle　筋肉	kidney　腎臓	appendix　虫垂
bone　骨	gallbladder　胆嚢	bladder　膀胱
joint　関節	pancreas　膵臓	uterus　子宮
lung　肺	duodenum　十二指腸	ovary　卵巣
heart　心臓	small intestine　小腸	vagina　腟
rib　肋骨		

PRACTICE Writing

イラストの（　）内に正しい部位名，
器官名を下から選んで入れましょう.

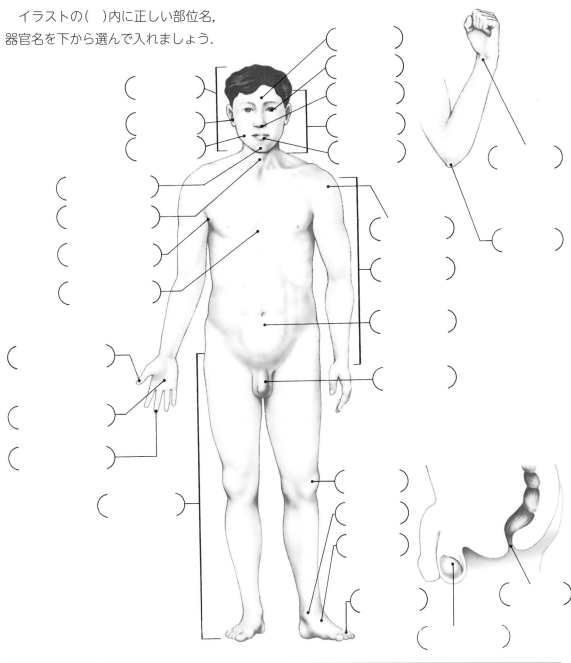

shoulder	chest	ankle	neck	forehead
foot	head	face	ear	testicles
thumb	cheek	toe	wrist	chin
nose	arm	leg	finger	palm
penis	mouth	elbow	armpit	abdomen
knee	eye	anus		

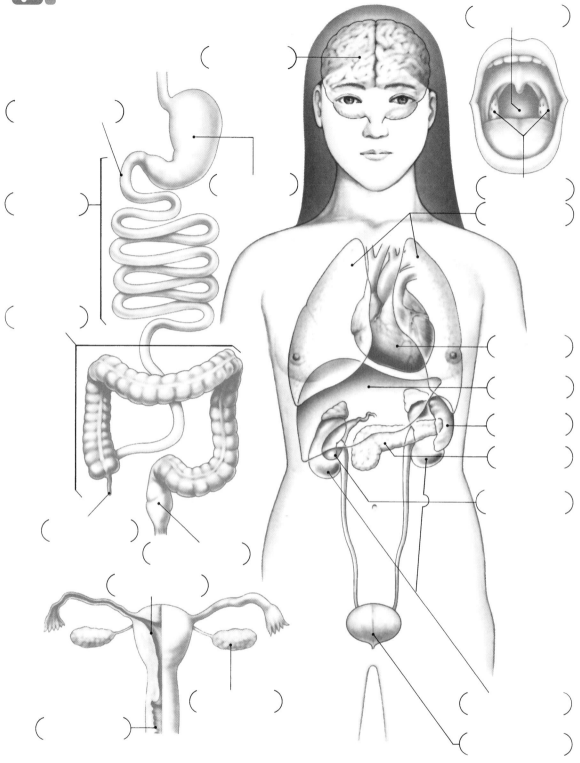

brain	liver	small intestine	large intestine
lungs	pancreas	bladder	appendix
duodenum	vagina	gallbladder	tonsils
ovary	uterus	heart	kidneys
rectum	stomach	spleen	throat

📖 PRACTICE Role Play

　2人一組になって，看護師役と患者役を決めます．

　看護師役は，患者に名前，症状，いつ頃からそうなったか，だんだん悪くなっているかなどを質問して，Aのカードの空欄をうめてください．患者役は，Bのカードにある外国人になったつもりで看護師の質問に答えてください．

　カードに記入し終わったら役割を交代して，患者役は今度はCのカードに記載された外国人になって繰り返し練習しましょう．

A：

氏名＿＿＿＿＿＿＿＿＿＿＿＿＿＿＿＿＿

1. どうしましたか？

＿＿＿＿＿＿＿＿＿＿＿＿＿＿＿＿＿＿＿

＿＿＿＿＿＿＿＿＿＿＿＿＿＿＿＿＿＿＿

2. それはいつ始まりましたか？＿＿＿＿＿＿＿＿

3. それは，（○をつけてください）

だんだん	大きく	
どんどん	悪く	なっている

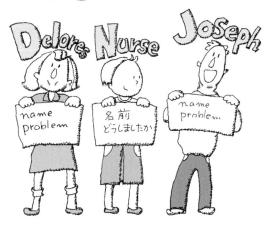

B :

> **Name :** *Delores Sato*
>
> **Problem :** *I have a lump in my right breast.*
> *I noticed it one month ago.*
> *It's getting bigger gradually.*

C :

> **Name :** *Joseph Robalino*
>
> **Problem :** *I hurt my ankle playing baseball.*
> *I hurt it yesterday.*
> *The pain is getting worse quickly.*

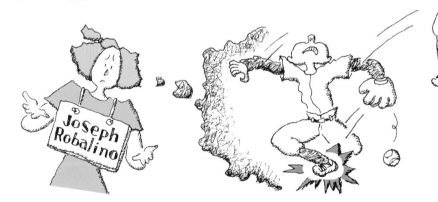

lump：しこり　　notice：気づく　　month：月　　get bigger：大きくなる
get worse：悪くなる

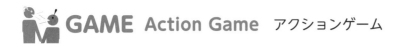 **GAME** Action Game アクションゲーム

先生が皆さんにある動作をするように指示しますから，皆さんはその指示に従って動作をします．

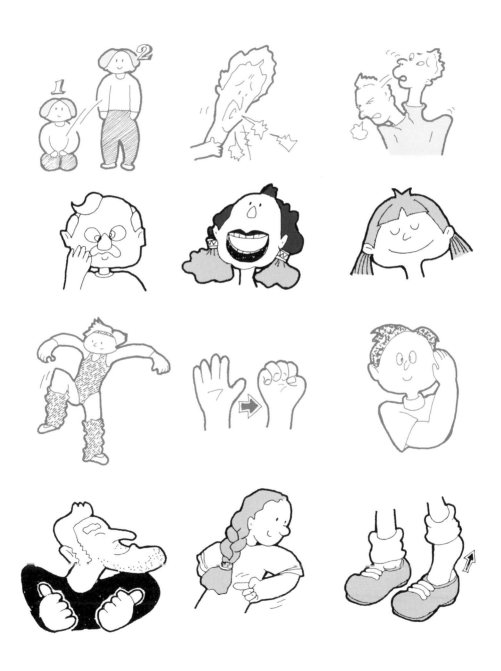

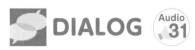

Unit 8 Have you ever had any serious illnesses?

🗨 DIALOG (Audio 31)

Masako : I'd like to ask you some questions about your medical history.

Mr. Lee : All right.

Masako : Have you ever had any serious illnesses?

Mr. Lee : I had asthma 15 years ago.

Masako : Do you have any allergies?

Mr. Lee : I'm allergic to cats and horses.

Masako : Are you allergic to any medication?

Mr. Lee : Yes, I'm allergic to penicillin.

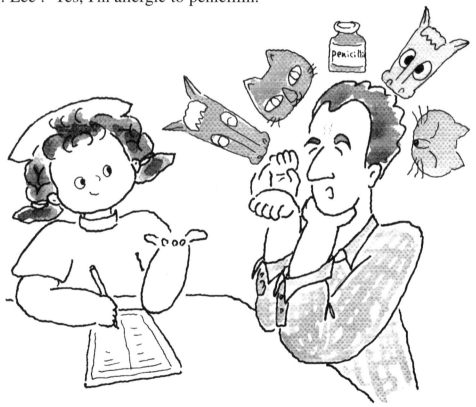

---

ever：今までに　　serious：重い，深刻な　　illness：病気　　medical history：病歴
asthma：喘息　　allergy：アレルギー　　be allergic to〜：〜にアレルギーがある
medication：薬物　　penicillin：ペニシリン

☑ CHECKPOINT

●病歴の尋ね方を覚えましょう.

1. 今までに重い病気をしたことがありますか.

   Have you ever had any serious illnesses?
   Have you ever been seriously ill?

   　Yes, I have.／No, I haven't.

2. その病気は何でしたか.

   What was the disease?

   　Breast cancer.

3. いつからそうなりましたか.

   When did it first start?

   それはいつでしたか.

   When was it?

   　Seven years ago.

4. 心臓病にかかっていますか(心臓病で苦しんでいますか).

   Do you suffer from heart disease?

   　Yes, I do.／No, I don't.

5. アレルギーはありますか.

   Do you have any allergies?

   　Yes, I do.／No, I don't.

6. どんなアレルギーですか.

   What allergies do you have?

   　I'm allergic to house-dust.

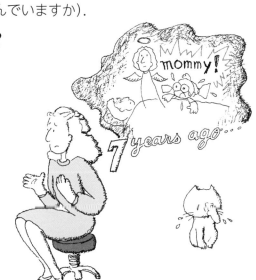

---

ill：病気にかかって 　disease：重病, 疾患, 〜病 　cancer：癌 　suffer from〜：〜(病気)に
かかっている, 〜で苦しんでいる 　house-dust：ハウスダスト

7. 薬に対するアレルギーはありますか.

Are you allergic to any medication?

Yes. I'm allergic to <u>penicillin.</u>／No. I'm not.

●時の表現を覚えましょう. Audio 33

今日	today		
昨日	yesterday	明日	tomorrow
一昨日	the day before yesterday	明後日	the day after tomorrow
3日前	3 days ago	3日後	3 days from now
先週	last week	来週	next week
先々週	the week before last	再来週	the week after next
3週間前	3 weeks ago	3週間後	3 weeks from now
去年	last year	来年	next year
一昨年	the year before last	再来年	the year after next
5年前	5 years ago	5年後	5 years from now

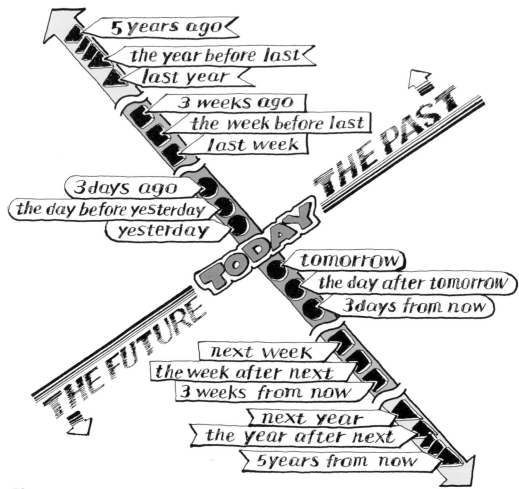

brain disease　脳の病気

lung disease　肺の病気

stomach disorder　胃の病気

intestinal disorder　腸の病気

kidney disease　腎臓病（疾患）

heart disease　心臓病（疾患）

liver disease　肝臓病（疾患）

mental disorder　心の病気

cancer　癌

tumor　腫瘍

hypertension　高血圧

duodenal ulcer　十二指腸潰瘍

gastric ulcer　胃潰瘍

anemia　貧血

tonsillitis　扁桃腺炎

appendicitis　虫垂炎

gallstone　胆石

cystitis　膀胱炎

vaginitis　腟炎

diabetes mellitus　糖尿病

asthma　喘息

rheumatoid arthritis

　　　　　　関節リウマチ

myoma of the uterus　子宮筋腫

cataract　白内障

glaucoma　緑内障

fracture　骨折

sprain　ねんざ

dislocation　脱臼

damaged ligament　靭帯損傷

gout　痛風

herniated disc　椎間板ヘルニア

tuberculosis　結核

pleurisy　胸膜炎

pneumonia　肺炎

bronchitis　気管支炎

allergy　アレルギー

eczema　湿疹

contact dermatitis　接触性皮膚炎

atopic dermatitis　アトピー性皮膚炎

hives　じん麻疹

infectious disease　感染症

common cold　軽いかぜ，鼻かぜ

hepatitis　肝炎

athlete's foot　足白癬（水虫）

measles　麻疹（はしか）

German measles, rubella　風疹

chickenpox　水痘

mumps　流行性耳下腺炎（おたふくかぜ）

pertussis　百日咳

roseola　突発性発疹（小児バラ疹）

STD（sexually transmitted disease）　性感染症

　HIV（human immunodeficiency virus）

　　　　　　　　　　ヒト免疫不全ウイルス

　AIDS（acquired immunodeficiency syndrome）

　　　　　　　　エイズ，後天性免疫不全症候群

syphilis　梅毒

herpes　疱疹（ヘルペス）

gonorrhea　淋病

📖 PRACTICE Writing

1. 1）〜 5）の文の空欄部分を①〜⑤から選んで補い，文章を完成させましょう.

   ① diabetes mellitus　　　② hypertension　　　③ gastric ulcer

   ④ allergy　　　　　　　⑤ tuberculosis

1）A _____ is an ulcer in the wall of the stomach.

2）_____ is a disease characterized by excessive
   amounts of sugar in the blood and urine.

3）_____ means high blood pressure.

4）_____ is a highly communicable disease caused
   by the tubercle bacillus (bacteria) and affecting
   mainly the lungs.

5）An _____ is a reaction such as sneezing,
   runny nose, itching or skin rash to substances
   such as food, pollen, dust, etc.

2. 1の答えをクロスワードに書き込んで,
   正しいかどうか確かめてください.

gastric
ulcer

---

ulcer：潰瘍　　stomach：胃　　characterize：特徴づける, 特性を表す　　excessive：過度の
amount of〜：〜の量　　blood：血液　　urine：尿　　blood pressure：血圧
communicable：伝染性の　　caused by：〜によって起こる　　tubercle bacillus：結核菌
bacteria：細菌　　affect：侵す　　mainly：主に　　lung：肺　　reaction：反応
such as〜：〜のような　　sneezing：くしゃみ　　runny nose：鼻水　　itching：かゆみ
rash：発疹　　substances：物質　　pollen：花粉　　dust：ほこり

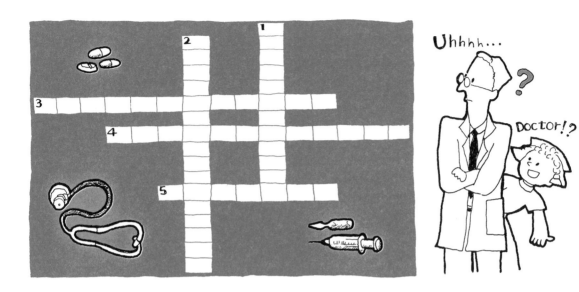

 ## PRACTICE Role Play

　2人一組になって，看護師役と患者役を決めます.

　看護師役は，患者に症状と病歴を質問してＡの内科予診票の空欄をうめてください. 患者役は，Ｂのカードにある外国人になったつもりで看護師の質問に答えてください. 内科予診票に記入し終わったら，役割を交代して，患者役は今度はＣのカードに記載された外国人になって繰り返し練習しましょう.

A:

内科予診票　　　　　　　　　　　　　　　　　　　　　年　　月　　日	

　氏名　　　　　　　　　　　　　　　　　　　　　　　男・女

1. どうしましたか.　＿＿＿＿＿＿＿＿＿＿＿＿＿＿＿＿＿＿＿

2. それはいつ始まりましたか.　＿＿＿＿＿＿＿＿＿＿＿＿＿＿

3. それは，（急に・徐々に）始まりましたか.

4. 痛みがありますか.（はい・いいえ）

5. どんな痛みですか.（激しい・鈍い刺すような）痛み

6. 大きな病気をしたことがありますか.（はい・いいえ）

　病名＿＿＿＿＿＿＿＿＿＿＿＿＿＿＿＿＿＿＿＿＿＿＿＿＿＿＿

7. その病気をしたのはいつですか.＿＿＿＿＿＿（か月・年）前

8. アレルギーがありますか.（はい・いいえ）

　アレルギーの種類＿＿＿＿＿＿＿＿＿＿＿＿＿＿＿＿＿＿＿＿＿

B :

Name : *Ruth Weinberg*

Problem : -*abdominal pain*
-*started yesterday*
-*started gradually*
-*severe pain*

Serious Past Illnesses or Problems :
-*no serious illnesses in the past*
-*allergic to penicillin*

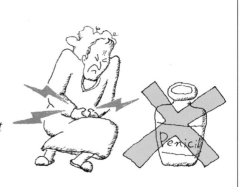

C :

Name : *Jennifer Newman*

Problem : -*high fever*
-*started 2 days ago*
-*started suddenly*
-*no other symptoms (no pain)*

Serious Past Illnesses or Problems:
-*heart disease*
-*started 5 years ago*
-*no allergy*

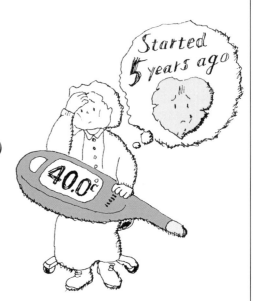

Started 5 years ago

40.0℃

---

abdominal pain：腹痛   severe pain：激痛   high fever：高熱   suddenly：突然
heart disease：心臓病

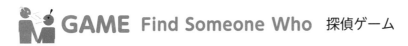

GAME Find Someone Who 探偵ゲーム

　下のリストの項目について，"Have you ever〜?"を使ってクラスメートに質問し，該当する人の名前をリストに書き込んでいきます．リストを全部うめたらゴールです．

Find someone who 〜   Name

　-has been to a foreign country.　　　　　　　_____

　-has ridden a roller coaster.　　　　　　　　_____

　-has eaten Indian food.　　　　　　　　　　_____

　-has had a part-time job.　　　　　　　　　_____

　-has knit a sweater.　　　　　　　　　　　_____

　-has seen a recent Disney movie.　　　　　　_____

　-has owned a pet.　　　　　　　　　　　　_____

　-has flown in an airplane.　　　　　　　　　_____

　-has stayed up all night without sleeping.　　_____

　-has gone skiing.　　　　　　　　　　　　_____

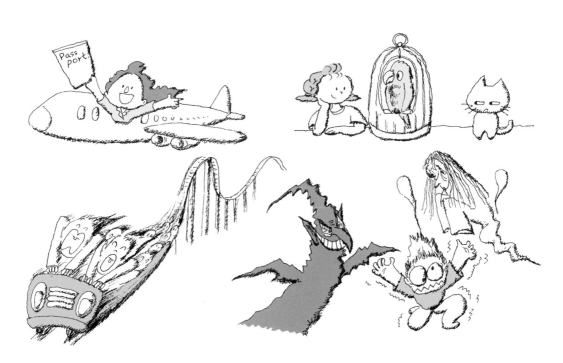

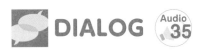

Unit 9 Take one tablet, four times a day.

DIALOG Audio 35

Masako : Your medicine is ready. This is cold medicine.

Take this for three days.

Mrs. Eisenberg : How often should I take it?

Masako : Take two tablets, three times a day after meals.

Mrs. Eisenberg : Two tablets, three times a day after meals.

Masako : That's right. Take them with a full glass of water.

Take care.

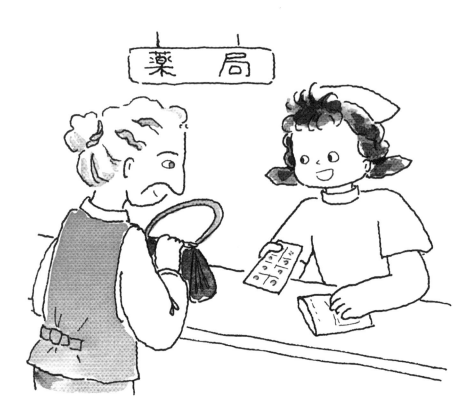

---

take：服用する　　tablet：錠剤　　cold medicine：かぜ薬　　how often〜：どのくらい(の頻度で)　　meal：食事　　a full glass of water：コップいっぱいの水　　take care：お大事に

☑ CHECKPOINT

●薬の服用に関する表現を覚えましょう.

1. お薬の用意ができています.

   Your medicine is ready.

   お薬をどうぞ.

   Here is your medicine.

2. この錠剤は食後に飲んでください.

   Take these tablets after meals.

3. 1日3回, 毎食後に飲んでください.

   Take this three times a day after each meal.

4. 寝る前に5mL飲んでください(水薬の場合).

   Take 5 mL before going to sleep.

   ＊薬のびんに数字の表示がない場合は, 目盛りを指し示しながら
   "Take this much." と言ってもよい.

5. これは外用のみのお薬です.

   This medicine is for external use only.

6. 肛門から坐薬を入れてください.

   You have to insert the suppository in your anus.
   You have to put the suppository into your anus.

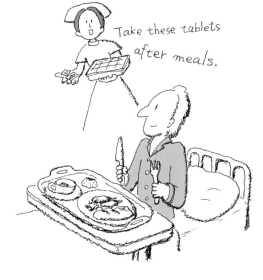

---

ready：用意ができて　　go to sleep：寝る　　external use：外用　　insert A in B：B に A を挿入する　　anus：肛門　　put A into B：B に A を入れる　　suppository：坐薬

7. 1日3〜4回，噴霧してください.

Use this spray three or four times a day.

8. 痛いときに飲んでください.

Take this when you have <u>pain</u>.

9. この軟膏を患部にぬってください.

Apply this ointment to the affected area.

●頻度の聞き方と答え方を覚えましょう. **Audio 37**

Q： How often do you <u>eat meat</u>?

A： 毎日　　　　　　　　　every day

　　1日に1回　　　　　　once a day

　　1週間に2回　　　　　twice a week

　　1か月に3回　　　　　three times a month

　　1年に4回　　　　　　four times a year

　　1時間ごとに1回　　　once every hour

　　2週間ごとに1回　　　once every two weeks

　　6か月ごとに1回　　　once every six months

　　3時間ごとに　　　　　every three hours

　　1日おきに　　　　　　every other day

　　全然〜しない　　　　　never

　　ほとんど〜しない　　　seldom

　　ときどき〜する　　　　sometimes

　　よく〜する　　　　　　very often

　　いつも〜する　　　　　always

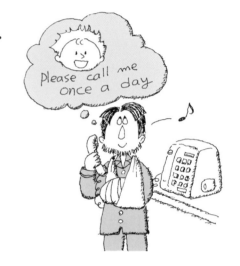

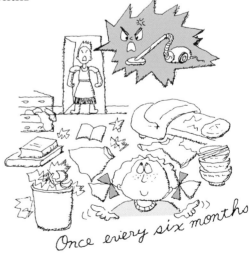

spray：スプレー　　apply：ぬる　　ointment：軟膏　　affected area：患部

●Internal use medicine（内服薬）

pill	錠剤，丸薬	powdered medicine	散剤，粉薬
tablet	錠剤	granular medicine	顆粒
capsule	カプセル	syrup	シロップ
liquid medicine	水薬	throat lozenge (troche)	トローチ

●External use medicine（外用薬）

cream	クリーム，ぬり薬	inhaler	吸入薬
ointment	軟膏	gargle	含嗽薬
suppository	坐薬	nose drops	点鼻薬
spray	スプレー	eye drops	点眼薬
plaster	貼付薬		

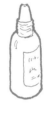

●Types of medicine（薬効別）

anti-pyretics (fever suppressant)	解熱剤	antibiotics	抗菌薬
cough medicine	鎮咳薬	laxatives	便秘薬
pain-killer	鎮痛薬	medicine for diarrhea	止痢薬
sleeping pills	睡眠薬	salve for itching	かゆみ止め

●Other treatment（その他）

injection	注射	blood transfusion	輸血
drip infusion	点滴		

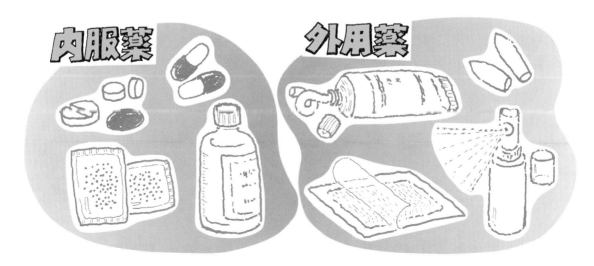

内服薬　外用薬

✏ PRACTICE Matching

1～13 の英文とそれに合った a～m の日本語を線で結びましょう.

1. ～ times a day

2. for ～ days

3. take ～ tablets

4. before each meal

5. after each meal

6. between meals

7. before breakfast and dinner

8. after breakfast and lunch

9. after every meal and before
   going to sleep

10. before going to sleep

11. every ～ hours

12. after breakfast and before
    going to sleep

13. follow your doctor's instructions

a. 毎食後と寝る前

b. 朝，夕食前

c. 医師の指示通りに

d. 1 日に～回

e. 朝食後と寝る前

f. ～時間ごとに

g. 毎食前

h. ～錠飲んでください

i. 食間

j. ～日分

k. 毎食後

l. 寝る前

m. 朝，昼食後

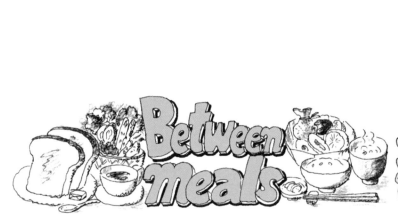

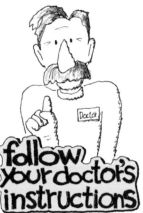

every～（数）：～（数）ごとに　　follow：従う　　instruction：指示

PRACTICE Listening

Audio を聞いて，下の薬袋に必要事項を書き入れましょう.

1)

```
──── 内用薬 ────
                    様
_____
   用法  1日   回   日分
        ┌ 散剤 _____ 包 ┐
        │ 錠剤 ___色___ 錠 │
  1回に │     ___色___   │ 服用
        │     ___色___   │
        │ カプセル ___色___ 個 │
        └     ___色___   ┘
  ＊毎食前      ＊食後と寝る前
  ＊毎食後      ＊寝る前
  ＊食間        ＊約   時間ごと
  ＊朝夕食前    ＊朝夕食後と寝る前
  ＊朝昼食後    ＊医師の指示通り
       ──── 令和  年 月 日 ────
```

2)

```
──── 内用薬 ────
                    様
_____
   用法  1日   回   日分
        ┌ 散剤 _____ 包 ┐
        │ 錠剤 ___色___ 錠 │
  1回に │     ___色___   │ 服用
        │     ___色___   │
        │ カプセル ___色___ 個 │
        └     ___色___   ┘
  ＊毎食前      ＊食後と寝る前
  ＊毎食後      ＊寝る前
  ＊食間        ＊約   時間ごと
  ＊朝夕食前    ＊朝夕食後と寝る前
  ＊朝昼食後    ＊医師の指示通り
       ──── 令和  年 月 日 ────
```

PRACTICE Writing

下の薬袋を見て，用法の説明文を書いてみましょう.

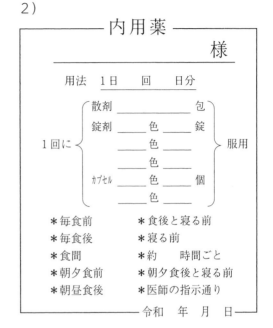

```
──── 内用薬 ────
                    様
_____
   用法  1日 3 回 5 日分
        ┌ 散剤 ___1___ 包 ┐
        │ 錠剤 ___色___ 錠 │
  1回に │     ___色___   │ 服用
        │     ___色___   │
        │ カプセル 黄 色 2 個 │
        └     赤 色 1   ┘
  ＊毎食前      ＊食後と寝る前
  ＊毎食後      ＊寝る前
  ＊食間        ＊約   時間ごと
  ＊朝夕食前   ⊛朝夕食後と寝る前
  ＊朝昼食後    ＊医師の指示通り
       ──── 令和  年 月 日 ────
```

_____

_____

_____

_____

✏ PRACTICE Role Play

2人一組になって，看護師役と患者役を決めます.

看護師役は，Aの薬袋を見ながら患者に用法を説明してください. 患者役は，看護師の説明をよく聞いて，Cの質問の答えを書いてください. 説明がわからない時は自分から質問しましょう.

質問用紙に記入し終わったら役割を交代して，看護師役は今度はBの薬袋を見ながら説明してください.

A：

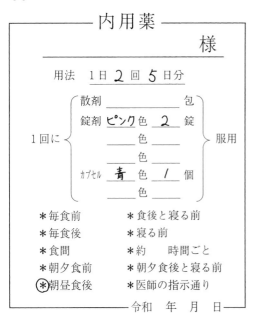

```
────── 内用薬 ──────
                              様
_____

    用法  1日 2 回 5 日分
        ┌ 散剤 _____ 包 ┐
        │ 錠剤 ピンク色 2 錠 │
  1回に  │    ____ 色 ____  ├ 服用
        │    ____ 色 ____  │
        │ カプセル 青 色 1 個 │
        └    ____ 色 ____ ┘

  ＊毎食前      ＊食後と寝る前
  ＊毎食後      ＊寝る前
  ＊食間        ＊約   時間ごと
  ＊朝夕食前    ＊朝夕食後と寝る前
  ⊛朝昼食後    ＊医師の指示通り
        ── 令和  年 月 日──
```

B：

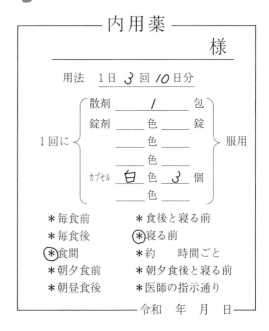

```
────── 内用薬 ──────
                              様
_____

    用法  1日 3 回 10 日分
        ┌ 散剤 ____ 1 ____ 包 ┐
        │ 錠剤 ____ 色 ____ 錠 │
  1回に  │    ____ 色 ____  ├ 服用
        │    ____ 色 ____  │
        │ カプセル 白 色 3 個 │
        └    ____ 色 ____ ┘

  ＊毎食前      ＊食後と寝る前
  ＊毎食後      ⊛寝る前
  ⊛食間        ＊約   時間ごと
  ＊朝夕食前    ＊朝夕食後と寝る前
  ＊朝昼食後    ＊医師の指示通り
        ── 令和  年 月 日──
```

C：

1. 何種類の薬？ _____

2. 薬の剤形，色，服用量は？ _____

   _____

3. 1日の服用回数は？ _____

4. いつ服用する？ _____

5. 服用期間は？ _____

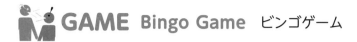 **GAME** Bingo Game　ビンゴゲーム

　下の各項目について，"How often do you~?" を使ってクラスメートに質問します．その回答を聞いて，該当する箇所に回答した人の名前を書き入れます．

　早く名前が5つ並んだ人が勝ちです．

A. How often

do you~?	everyday	very often	sometimes	seldom	never
-play tennis?					
-go to the movies?					
-clean your room?					
-eat rice for breakfast?					
-do a part-time job?					

B. How often

do you~?	everyday	very often	sometimes	seldom	never
-go to karaoke?					
-telephone your friend?					
-drink coffee?					
-cook dinner?					
-go to bed after midnight?					

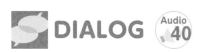

Unit 10 Let me make an appointment for your test.

◆DIALOG Audio 40

Mr. Ford : The doctor said I need to have a gastroscopy.

Masako : I see. Let me make an appointment for you. There's an
opening on Friday morning at 9:30. Can you come then?

Mr. Ford : I'm afraid I'm busy then.

Masako : Well, how about next Monday at 10:00?

Mr. Ford : Yes, I'm free then.

Masako : O.K. I'll put you down for Monday at 10:00. Don't eat or
drink anything after 9 p.m. on Sunday evening.

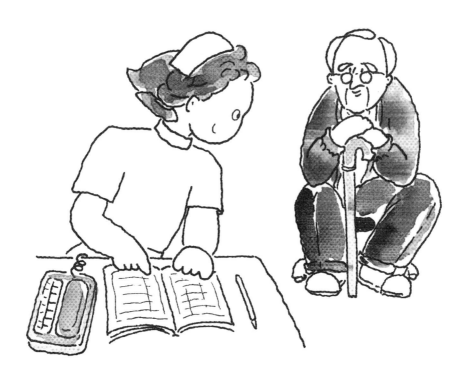

make an appointment for～：～の予約を取る　　test：検査　　gastroscopy：胃内視鏡検査
opening：あき，予約の入っていない　　be afraid：あいにく，すみませんが　　be busy：予定
が入っている　　how about～：～はどうですか　　be free：予定がない，あいている　　put～
down：書き入れる　　not～(動詞)anything：なにも～しない，全然～しない

☑ CHECKPOINT

● 予約の取り方を覚えましょう. Audio 41

1. 患者が予約をする場合：検査の予約をしたいのですが.

　　　I'd like to make an appointment for my test.

2. 看護師が患者のために予約をとる場合：検査の予約をしておきましょう.

Let me make an appointment for your test.

3. 来週の金曜日があいていますが, 来られますか.

There's an opening <u>next Friday</u>. Can you come on that day?

　　　Yes, I can.

　　　I'm afraid I'm busy then.（あいにくですが, その日は忙しいです）

　　　No. But I'm free on July third.（いいえ, でも7月3日ならあいています）

4. 別の日時を提案する場合：来週の月曜, 朝9時半はどうですか.

How about <u>next Monday at 9 : 30 in the morning</u>?

5. では, 9月10日の午後2時に予約をお取りしておきます.

I'll put you down for <u>September 10th, at 2 : 00</u>.

● 時間の表現を覚えましょう. Audio 42

four o'clock

four a.m.

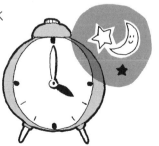

four p.m.

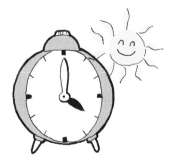

would like to～：～したい　　noon：正午　　midnight：夜中

three thirty
half past three

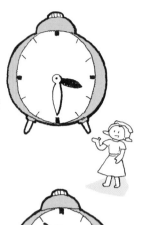

twelve noon

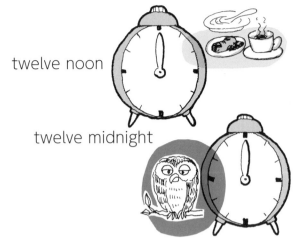

twelve midnight

eleven fifty-five
five to twelve
five minutes before twelve

six fifteen
quarter past six
fifteen after six

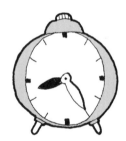

nine forty
twenty to ten
twenty minutes before ten

eight twenty-five

●検査に関する表現を覚えましょう. Audio 43

1. このカップに尿（便）を採ってきてください.

   Please collect your urine (stool) in this cup.

2. こちらでお待ちください.

   Please wait here.

3. こちらにお入りください.

   This way, please.

4. ここに横になってください.

   Please lie down here.

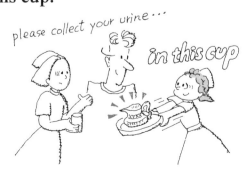

please collect your urine…

in this cup

5. うつ伏せ(あお向け，横向き)になってください.

   Please lie face down (face up／on your side).

6. 楽にしてください(力を抜いてください).

   Relax.

7. 拳をぎゅうっと握ってください.

   Make a fist and squeeze.

8. これを着てください.

   Please put this on.

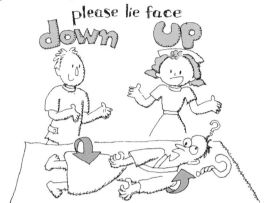

---

collect：採取する 　 urine：尿 　 stool：便 　 lie down：横になる
lie face down：うつ伏せになる 　 relax：楽にする，リラックスする 　 fist：拳
squeeze：強く握る 　 put~on：~を着る

MEDICAL TERMS Tests 　検査の言い方を覚えましょう. 　Audio 44

eye test 　視力検査

hearing test 　聴力検査

blood test 　血液検査

blood chemistry test 　血液生化学検査

urinalysis (urine test) 　尿検査

blood specimen collection 　採血

stool test 　便検査

fecal occult blood test 　便潜血検査

sputum test 　喀痰検査

electrocardiogram (ECG) 　心電図検査

gastroscopy 　胃内視鏡検査

colonoscopy 　大腸内視鏡検査

uterine cancer screening (pap test／pap smear) 　子宮癌検査

vaginal examination 　腟内診

rectal examination 　直腸診

electroencephalogram (EEG) 　脳波検査

angiography 　血管造影

barium enema 　バリウム注腸造影

upper (lower) GI (gastrointestinal) series

　上部(下部) 消化管撮影

ultrasound (echogram) 　超音波検査

X-ray examination 　X 線検査

CT (computed tomography)

　コンピュータ断層撮影

MRI (magnetic resonance imaging)

　磁気共鳴画像法

PRACTICE Listening

Audio の会話を聞いて, 時間を書き取りましょう.

1) ＿＿＿＿＿＿＿＿＿　　2) from＿＿＿＿to＿＿＿＿＿

3) ＿＿＿＿＿＿＿＿＿　　4) between＿＿＿＿and＿＿＿＿＿

5) ＿＿＿＿＿＿＿＿＿　　6) ＿＿＿＿＿＿＿＿＿

PRACTICE Role Play

2人一組になって, 看護師役と患者役を決めます.

看護師役は A のスケジュール表を見ながら, 電話をかけてきた患者と日時を調節して予約を取ります. 患者役は次頁 B, C のスケジュールを見ながら, 病院に電話をして診察の予約を取ります ("Hello. Sato Clinic. May I help you?" で始めてください).

予約が取れたら, 役割を交代して繰り返し練習しましょう.

A:

今週のスケジュール　4月

		AM 9:00	10:00	11:00	12:00	PM 1:00		3:00	4:00	5:00	備 考
月	10					お					あきなし
火	11					昼					あき 9:30a.m～10:30am
水	12					休					あき 10:00am～11:00am 3:15pm～4:00pm
木	13					み					午後あき
金	14										あき 3:45pmより

MEMO

佐藤クリニック

B :

Jessica Robinson のスケジュール

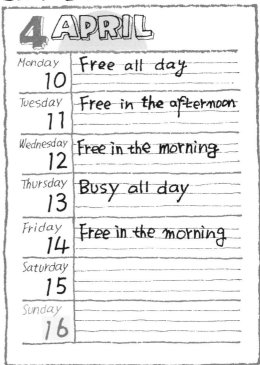

4 APRIL

Monday 10	Free in the morning
Tuesday 11	Busy all day
Wednesday 12	Busy all day
Thursday 13	Free in the afternoon
Friday 14	Free all day
Saturday 15	
Sunday 16	

C :

Brian Baker のスケジュール

4 APRIL

Monday 10	Free all day
Tuesday 11	Free in the afternoon
Wednesday 12	Free in the morning
Thursday 13	Busy all day
Friday 14	Free in the morning
Saturday 15	
Sunday 16	

GAME Pass It On 伝言ゲーム

　いくつかのチームに分かれ，チームごとに縦1列に並びます.

　先生が各列の先頭の学生に伝言文を言いますから，皆さんはスタートの合図で，ほかのチームに聞こえないように，前から順々にその言葉を伝えていきます．最後の人まで正しく伝えられたチームの勝ちです.

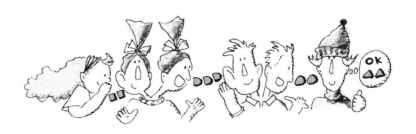

Your surgery will be tomorrow at 9 a.m.

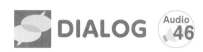

DIALOG

Masako : Your surgery will be tomorrow. Before your surgery, you have to sign this consent form. If you have a seal, please stamp your seal here.

Miss Jones : What time is my surgery tomorrow?

Masako : Your surgery will be at 9 a.m. This evening you cannot eat or drink anything.

Miss Jones : I see.

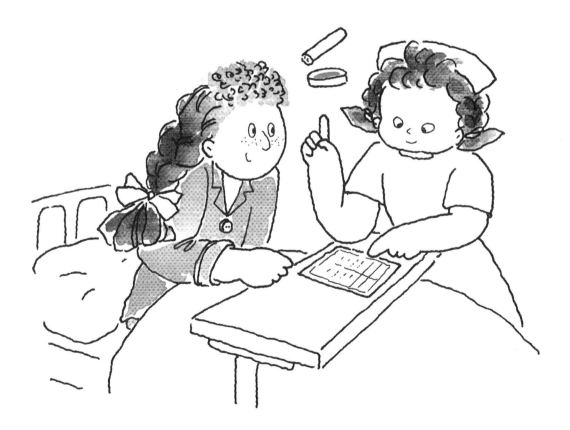

surgery：手術　　have to～：～しなければならない　　sign：署名する　　consent form：承
諾書　　seal：印鑑　　stamp：判を押す　　not～anything：何も～ない，全然～ない

CHECKPOINT 手術に関する表現を覚えましょう.

[**The day before surgery** 手術前夜]

1. 今日の夕食は流動食になります.

   You will have a liquid meal this evening.

2. 睡眠薬を飲んでください.

   Please take the sleeping pill.

3. お風呂に入ってください.

   Please take a bath.

4. ここに(この承諾書に)署名してください.

   Please sign here (this consent form).

5. ここに印鑑を押してください.

   Please stamp your seal here.

6. おなかの(体)毛を剃ります.

   Your abdominal area will be shaved.

   I have to shave your abdominal area.

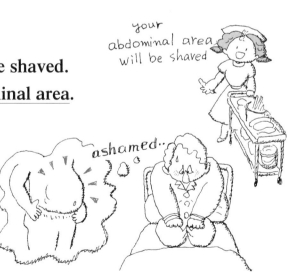

---

liquid meal：流動食　　sleeping pill：睡眠薬　　take a bath：風呂に入る　　abdominal area：おなかの部分　　shave：剃る

[**The day of surgery**　手術当日]

1. 浣腸をします.

   You will have to have an enema.

   トイレを済ませておいてください.

   You will have to go to the toilet.

2. カテーテルを膀胱に挿入し，手術後1，2日したら外します.

   **A catheter will be inserted into your bladder. It will be removed
   a day or two after your surgery.**

3. 胃管を鼻から挿入します.

   A gastric tube will be inserted through your nose.

4. 手術の30分くらい前に，鎮静薬が投与されます.

   About 30 minutes before surgery, you will be given a sedative.

5. 点滴静注をします.

   You will be put on an intravenous drip.

[**After surgery**　手術後]

1. 1週間後，医師が抜糸します.

   The doctor will remove your stitches a week from today.

2. もし痛むようでしたら，痛み止めを注射します(鎮痛薬を投与します).

   If you have pain, I will give you a shot for the pain (a pain-killer).

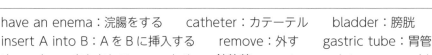

---

have an enema：浣腸をする　　catheter：カテーテル　　bladder：膀胱
insert A into B：AをBに挿入する　　remove：外す　　gastric tube：胃管
through：～をとおして　　sedative：鎮静薬　　put on an intravenous drip：点滴静注をする
stitches：縫合，糸　　shot：注射　　a pain-killer：鎮痛薬

●未来形の "be going to" と "will" の使い方を覚えましょう.

[be going to]　一般に自分の意思ですることを表現するとき

I am going to go shopping tomorrow.　（明日，買い物に行きます）

　　　　　　meet my friend tonight.　（今夜，友達に会います）

[will]　話し手の意思を述べるときにも使われるが，例のように，

　　　　自分の意思とはかかわりなく起こる未来の出来事を表現することができる.

The train will leave at 10:35 a.m.　（電車は午前 10 時 35 分に出ます）

The examination will be finished soon.　（検査はもうすぐ終わります）

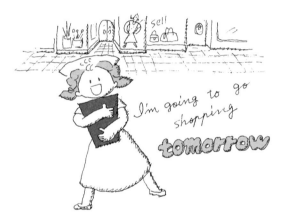

PRACTICE Speaking & Listening

　2 人一組になって交互に質問し，相手の答えを書き取りましょう.

1. What are you going to do next Sunday?

2. What will be your first class tomorrow?

3. When are you going to get your hair cut?

4. What time will your last class finish today?

5. What are you going to do after this class?

---

leave：出発する　　examination：検査　　finish：終わる

PRACTICE Writing & Speaking

2人一組になって，次の設定条件に合った会話文を完成してください．会話文が完成したら，お互いに役割を決めて会話の練習をしましょう．

●手術前日のオリエンテーションの内容

患者氏名：John Rogers
手術の日時：September 13, 20XX, 10:30 a.m.
手術の種類：Removal of gallbladder (cholecystectomy)　胆嚢摘出
手術前の必要処置：

　［手術前日］

1. sign a consent form
2. shave chest and abdominal area
3. take a bath
4. have a liquid meal
5. don't eat or drink anything after 9 p.m.
6. take a sleeping pill at 9 p.m.

　［手術当日朝］

1. go to the toilet
2. a catheter will be inserted into the bladder
3. a gastric tube will be inserted through the nose

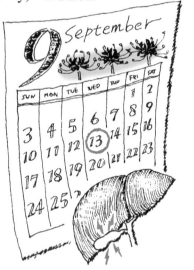

●完成すべき会話文　Audio 48

Nurse : Mr. Rogers, your surgery ＿＿＿＿＿＿ ＿＿＿＿＿＿ tomorrow.

　　　　Before your surgery, you ＿＿＿＿＿ ＿＿＿＿＿ ＿＿＿＿＿

　　　　＿＿＿＿＿ ＿＿＿＿＿ ＿＿＿＿＿. And ＿＿＿＿＿

　　　　＿＿＿＿＿ your seal here.

Patient : ＿＿＿＿＿ ＿＿＿＿＿ ＿＿＿＿＿ ＿＿＿＿＿ surgery?

Nurse : It's at 10:30 a.m.

　　　　Today I have to ＿＿＿＿＿ ＿＿＿＿＿ ＿＿＿＿＿

　　　　＿＿＿＿＿ ＿＿＿＿＿ ＿＿＿＿＿. Please ＿＿＿＿＿

　　　　＿＿＿＿＿ ＿＿＿＿＿.

This evening you will have _____ _____ _____.

Please don't _____ _____ _____ after 9:00 p.m.

Patient : I see.

Nurse : At 9:00 p.m., please take the _____ _____.

Patient : O.K.

Nurse : Tomorrow morning you will have to _____ _____ _____

_____.

A _____ will be _____ _____ your

_____ and a _____ _____ will be

_____ _____ _____.

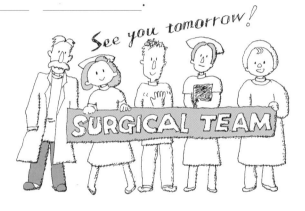

GAME BUZZ! バズゲーム

グループで輪になって座り，1～100 までの数字を順々に言っていきます．その際に，スペシャルナンバーを 1 つ決めておき，スペシャルナンバーが含まれている数字またはそのナンバーの倍数のところでは，数字を言う代わりに "BUZZ!" と言います．

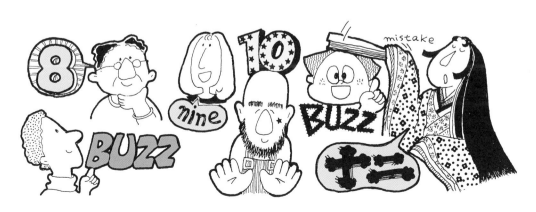

Unit 12 How are you feeling today?

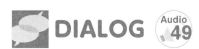

DIALOG Audio 49

Masako : Good morning, Mr. Robinson.

Mr. Robinson : Good morning.

Masako : How are you feeling today?

Mr. Robinson : Pretty good.

Masako : Please take your temperature. Yesterday, how many times did you move your bowels and urinate?

Mr. Robinson : I moved my bowels twice and urinated 5 times.

Masako : Did you have a good appetite or a poor appetite?

Mr. Robinson : I had a good appetite. I ate 3/4 of my meals.

Masako : All right. Let's see, what's your temperature?

Mr. Robinson : It's 36.5 ℃.

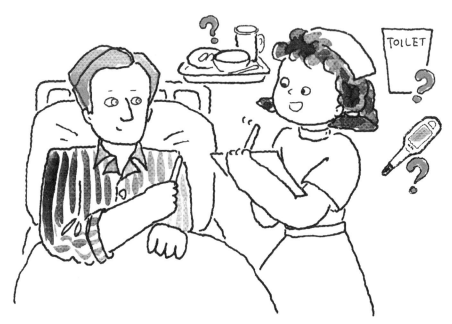

How are you feeling? : 気分はいかがですか　　pretty : とても　　take one's temperature : 体温を計る　　move one's bowels : 排便する　　urinate : 排尿する　　good (poor)
appetite : 食欲がある(ない)　　let's see : えーと　　℃ : degrees Celsius (centigrade)

☑ CHECKPOINT 入院患者によくする質問を覚えましょう. Audio 50

1. 気分はいかがですか.

   How are you?

   How are you feeling today?

   > Fine, thank you.
   >
   > Pretty good. (なかなかいいです)
   >
   > Not so good. (あまりよくありません)
   >
   > Terrible. (とても悪いです)

2. どうしたんですか.

   What's the problem?

   > I couldn't sleep very well. (よく眠れませんでした)

3. 脈(血圧)を計ります.

   I have to take your pulse (blood pressure).

4. 体温を計ります.

   I'm going to take your temperature.

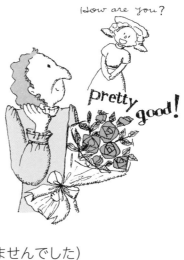

5. 採血します.

   I need a blood sample (a sample of your blood).

   I need to take some blood.

6. このコップに尿(便)をとってください.

   Please put a urine (stool) sample in this cup.

7. 昨日, 排便は何回ありましたか.

   Yesterday, how many times did you move your bowels?

   > Once. (1回)／Twice. (2回)／Three times. (3回)

---

terrible：とても悪い　　pulse：脈　　blood pressure：血圧　　sample：サンプル
urine：尿　　stool：便

8. 食欲はありましたか.

Did you have a good appetite?

Yes, I did.／No, I didn't.

So so.（まあまあでした）

9. 体温は何度ですか.

What's your temperature?

My temperature is normal.

It's 38.5℃.

10. ふだんの食事内容はどんなものですか.

What is your usual diet?

I eat lots of fruits and vegetables.（果物，野菜をよくとります）

I prefer fish to meat dishes.（肉よりも魚料理を好んで食べます）

I usually don't eat balanced meals.

　（ふだんあまりバランスのよい食事をしていません／偏食です）

I'm a vegetarian.（ベジタリアンです）

●**Fractions**　分数の読み方を覚えましょう. Audio **51**

1/2　one-half あるいは a half

1/3　one-third

1/4　one-fourth あるいは one (a) -quarter

1/5　one-fifth

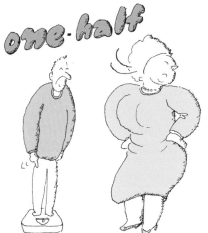

分子が 2 以上の数になると，分母に s をつけます.

2/3　two-thirds

3/4　three-fourths あるいは three-quarters

so so：まあまあ　　diet：食事内容，食習慣　　lots of：たくさんの	
prefer A to B：B より A を好む　　dish：料理　　balanced meal：バランスのとれた食事	
fraction：分数	

✏️ PRACTICE Listening

Audio を聞いて，分数を書き取りましょう．

1） _____   2） _____   3） _____

4） _____   5） _____   6） _____

✏️ PRACTICE Writing

次の分数の読み方を書いてみましょう．

1） 1/4 _____   2） 1/2 _____   3） 1/3 _____

4） 2/3 _____   5） 3/5 _____   6） 3/4 _____

✏️ PRACTICE Speaking & Listening

　次の質問は，看護師が入院してきた患者に，あるいは訪室したときによくする質問です．2人一組になって交互に質問し，相手の答えを書き取りましょう．

1．How are you feeling?

2．Do you have a good appetite?

3．What is your usual diet?

4．Yesterday, how many times did you urinate?

5．What time do you usually go to bed and get up?

6．How tall are you?

7．How much do you weigh?

8．Do you have any allergies?

9．How often do you drink alcohol?

10．Do you smoke?

---

get up：起きる　　tall：身長がある　　weigh：体重がある　　allergy：アレルギー
alcohol：酒　　smoke：たばこを吸う

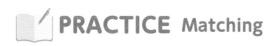

PRACTICE Matching

絵を見て，看護師が患者に何と言っているのかを，下の文章から選んでください．

1. It's time to take your medicine.
2. Your intravenous drip is finished.
3. Do you have a headache?
4. Supper is ready.
5. Shall I open the window?
6. Please wait. The doctor will see you soon.
7. Don't smoke here, please.
8. I want to take your blood pressure.
9. Did you sleep well last night?

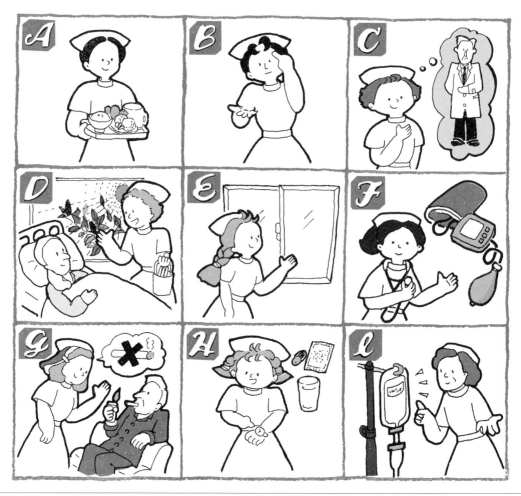

medicine：薬　　intravenous drip：点滴　　supper：夕食　　shall I 〜?：〜しましょうか
see：診察する　　blood pressure：血圧

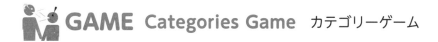

GAME Categories Game カテゴリーゲーム

4人ずつくらいのグループを作ります.

先生が単語の種類と先頭文字を言いますから，皆さんはそれに当てはまる英単語を見つけ出します. 早く見つけたグループから答えを言っていき，答えた単語の数でポイントを競います. カテゴリーは，Departments (p.23参照)，Symptoms (p.34, 35)，External Body Parts (p.42)，Internal Body Parts (p.42)，Diseases (p.51)，Tests (p.67)です.

出題例）カテゴリー：symptoms　　先頭文字：C

解答例）cough／cramps／constipation／chest pain

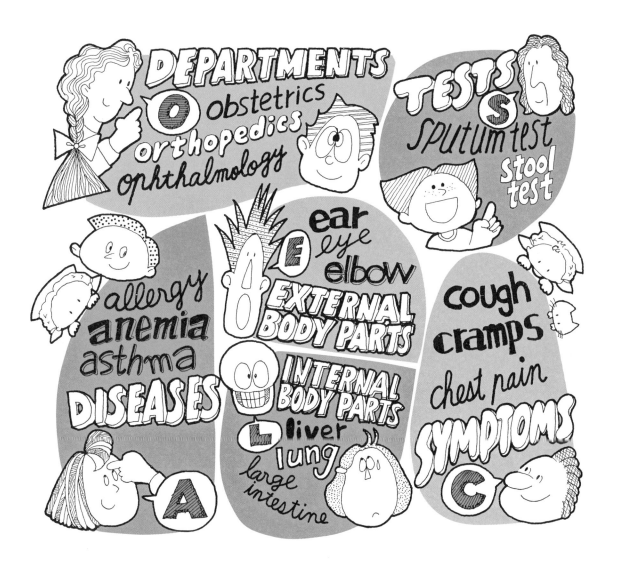

WORD LIST

A

a cup of 〜 1杯の〜 17

a few 少しの, 2, 3の 32

a full glass of 〜 コップいっぱいの〜 56

abdomen 腹 42

abdominal area おなかの部分 71, 74

abdominal pain 腹痛 34, 54

accounting 会計 28

address 住所 16, 25

affect 侵す 52

affected area 患部 58

age 年齢 25

AIDS(acquired immunodeficiency syndrome)
エイズ；後天性免疫不全症候群 51

alcohol 酒 79

allergy アレルギー 48, 51, 54, 79
be allergic to 〜 〜にアレルギーがある

alone 1人で 13

amount of 〜 〜の量 52

anemia 貧血 51

anesthesiology 麻酔科 23

angiography 血管造影 67

ankle 足首, くるぶし 42, 46

anti-pyretics 解熱剤 59

antibiotics 抗菌薬 59

anus 肛門 42, 57

apartment アパート 18

appendicitis 虫垂炎 51

appendix 虫垂 42

appetite 食欲 34, 76, 78
appetite loss 食欲不振
good appetite 食欲がある
poor appetite 食欲がない

apply (薬を)ぬる 58

appointment 予約 64, 65
make an appointment for 〜 〜の予約を取る

arm 腕 35, 42

armpit 腋窩 42

asthma 喘息 48, 51

athlete's foot 足白癬(水虫) 51

atopic dermatitis アトピー性皮膚炎 51

B

bacillus 桿状細菌 52

back 背中 40, 42

backache 背中の痛み, 腰痛 34, 35

bacteria 細菌 52

balanced meal バランスのとれた食事 78

bank 銀行 28

barium enema バリウム注腸造影 67

be afraid あいにく, すみませんが 64, 65

be allergic to 〜 〜にアレルギーがある 48-50, 54

be born 生まれる 12, 15

be busy 予定が入っている 64, 65

be free 予定がない, あいている 64, 65

be from 〜の出身である 11, 12

birthplace 出生地 12, 25

bladder 膀胱 37, 42, 72

bleeding 出血 34, 35

blood 血液 52, 77
— chemistry test 血液生化学検査 67
— lab 血液検査室 28
— pressure 血圧 52, 77, 80
— sample 血液検体 77
— specimen collection 採血 67
— stool 血便 34
— test 血液検査 67
— transfusion 輸血 59

bone 骨 42

bowel 腸(腸の一部) 76
move one's bowels 排便する

brain 脳 42

brain disease 脳の病気 51

breast 乳房 42, 46

breast cancer 乳癌 49

bronchitis 気管支炎 51

burping げっぷ 34

buttock 殿部 42

C

calf ふくらはぎ 42